# THE
# NEXUS
## NURSING FRAMEWORK

*Building the Workforce
our Communities Deserve*

# SHERRI JOHNSON
DNP, MPA, RN, FADLN, FAAN

Cover and interior formatting by KUHN Design Group | kuhndesigngroup.com

The NEXUS Nursing Framework™ is a trademark of The Johnson Consulting Group LLC. Trademark registration pending.

ISBN: 979-8-218-88591-5 (paperback)
ISBN: 979-8-218-93470-5 (hardcover)

Printed in the United States of America First Edition, 2026

"This book is a game changer and a clarion call to action! At a time when the nursing workforce crisis threatens the very foundation of the healthcare system, this work offers a bold and visionary blueprint for change. By reframing the challenge as an infrastructure imperative, Dr. Johnson charts a path that connects K-12 pathways, higher education learning and federal workforce policy into a unified, sustainable solution. But the unique approach that she uses is not just a framework. It is the beginning of a movement to secure the future of nursing and, ultimately, the health of our nation. Every educator, policymaker, and healthcare leader should read this book and join forces in an effort to build the workforce we so desperately need...before it's too late!"

**Ernest J. Grant, PhD, DSc(h), RN, FAAN**
Former President—American Nurses Association

"As someone who has worked both in federal policy and nursing leadership, I recognize the gaps Dr. Johnson identifies in The NEXUS Nursing Framework. For too long, Black and underrepresented communities have been excluded from nursing pathways not due to lack of interest, but due to infrastructure barriers—disconnected funding streams, limited clinical capacity, and misaligned educational policies. However, this framework provides the roadmap we need to build a more equitable nursing workforce infrastructure. It is both practical and forward thinking in its scope. Nursing is our country's pathway to health equity and a well diversified nursing workforce will benefit all in our society."

**—Sheldon D. Fields, PhD, RN, CRNP,**
**FNP-BC, AACRN, FAANP, FNAP, FADLN, FAAN**
14th President & CEO, National Black Nurses Association
Former Robert Wood Johnson Foundation Health Policy Fellow (2009)

Written by Dr. Sherri Johnson, *The Nexus Nursing Framework*™ offers a clear and comprehensive examination of one of nursing's most pressing challenges: building and sustaining a workforce capable of meeting today's needs—both domestically and globally. The nursing profession has long recognized that efforts to sustain the workforce, historically and in modern times, have fallen short.

Across its chapters, this book thoughtfully examines the factors that have contributed to—or distracted from—the development of a high-quality nursing workforce. Dr. Johnson brings critical insight to why previous workforce strategies have been less successful and moves the conversation forward by identifying solutions grounded in evidence, policy, and practice. Importantly, she offers strategies and policy recommendations that are not merely aspirational, but practical and actionable for individual nurses, leaders, and policymakers alike.

**Rebecca M. Patton, DNP, RN, CNOR, FAAN**
Past President, American Nurses Association

*The NEXUS Nursing Framework* brings timely attention to nursing education capacity as a critical infrastructure issue, skillfully connecting workforce shortages to investment decisions and the persistent challenge of misaligned incentives. With vivid real-world stories drawn from the author's experience as a nurse, leader, and mentor, the book offers both candor and compassion in its diagnosis of systemic breakdowns. Its emphasis on structural equity—especially the increasingly vital role of digital equity—reminds us that sustainable workforce solutions must be built on inclusive policy and practice. NEXUS is a comprehensive and well-informed perspective that invites leaders and policymakers to engage deeply with the realities shaping nursing today."

**Olga Yakusheva, PhD**, Economist, Professor,
Johns Hopkins School of Nursing, Johns Hopkins Business of Health/ HBHI
Johns Hopkins Bloomberg Center

# Contents

Preface . . . . . . . . . . . . . . . . . . . . . . . . . . . . . . . . . . . . 7

Acknowledgments . . . . . . . . . . . . . . . . . . . . . . . . . . . . 11

## PART I: THE UNTOLD STORY OF THE NURSING WORKFORCE CRISIS

1. The Nursing Workforce Crisis Is an Infrastructure Issue, Not a Shortage Problem . . . . . . . . . . . . . . . . . . . . . . . . 17

2. Why Our Current System Fails . . . . . . . . . . . . . . . . . . 25

3. The NEXUS Nursing Framework™ . . . . . . . . . . . . . . . 29

4. What K–12 Educators See That Policymakers Miss . . . . . 35

5. The Power of Community . . . . . . . . . . . . . . . . . . . . . . 43

6. What Nurses See . . . . . . . . . . . . . . . . . . . . . . . . . . . . 51

7. Higher Education and Clinical Capacity . . . . . . . . . . . . 61

## PART II: THE SYSTEMS THAT SHAPE US

8. Adult Learners and Working Students . . . . . . . . . . . . . 75

9. WIOA and Nursing Education . . . . . . . . . . . . . . . . . . 85

10. Title VIII . . . . . . . . . . . . . . . . . . . . . . . . . . . . . . . . 97

11. HRSA and Federal Levers . . . . . . . . . . . . . . . . . . . . 107

12. State Innovation . . . . . . . . . . . . . . . . . . . . . . . . . . . 119

## PART III: MAKING IT REAL

13. Cross-Sector Collaboration . . . . . . . . . . . . . . . . . . . . . . . . 133

14. The New Workforce Ecosystem . . . . . . . . . . . . . . . . . . . . 149

15. Families, Communities, & Faith Institutions as
    Workforce Builders . . . . . . . . . . . . . . . . . . . . . . . . . . . . 159

16. Leadership for the Next Generation . . . . . . . . . . . . . . . . 171

17. Policy Recommendations . . . . . . . . . . . . . . . . . . . . . . . . . 181

18. Nursing as Calling, Infrastructure, and Shared
    Responsibility . . . . . . . . . . . . . . . . . . . . . . . . . . . . . . . . . 191

Appendix A: Strengthening Career and Technical
    Education for the 21st Century Act . . . . . . . . . . . . . . . 203

Appendix B: Acronyms and Definitions . . . . . . . . . . . . . . . 207

Appendix C: Summary of The NEXUS Nursing
    FrameworkTM . . . . . . . . . . . . . . . . . . . . . . . . . . . . . . . . 211

Appendix D: Crosswalk of Federal Levers
    (Perkins V, WIOA, Title VIII, HRSA) . . . . . . . . . . . . . 215

Appendix E: Critical Breakdown Points in Nursing
    Pathways: A Stage-by-Stage Infrastructure Analysis . . . 217

Appendix F: Policy Recommendations by Sector . . . . . . . 221

Appendix G: Economic Impact Calculation
    Methodology . . . . . . . . . . . . . . . . . . . . . . . . . . . . . . . . . 225

Appendix H: References & Resources . . . . . . . . . . . . . . . . 229

Index . . . . . . . . . . . . . . . . . . . . . . . . . . . . . . . . . . . . . . . . . . 239

About the Author . . . . . . . . . . . . . . . . . . . . . . . . . . . . . . . 243

# Preface

For decades, conversations about the nursing workforce have often been framed around a familiar and urgent phrase: *the nursing shortage*. The phrase has served an important purpose, drawing attention to real challenges and prompting critical research, policy discussions, and investments. Within the nursing profession, workforce challenges have long been understood as cyclical and deeply connected to issues of safety, burnout, working conditions, and moral distress.

Outside of nursing, however, these challenges are often interpreted through a narrower operational lens—focused on recruitment, incentives, or short-term fixes—without full consideration of the broader structural conditions that shape nursing pathways.

Alongside this professional framing, significant efforts have been made to articulate the economic value of nursing and its contribution to health systems, communities, and national well-being. Together, these perspectives underscore that nursing is not only essential to care delivery, but foundational to how health systems function.

This book begins from a related, but broader premise: the nursing workforce is infrastructure.

Like transportation systems, broadband, or clean water, nursing infrastructure determines whether communities function, whether public health systems can respond to crises, and whether families can access care when it matters most. When that infrastructure is strong, societies are resilient. When it weakens, the consequences ripple far beyond hospitals—into schools, workplaces, and entire regions.

Despite nursing's central role, the systems responsible for educating, supporting, and sustaining nurses have developed along largely separate tracks. Education, workforce development, healthcare delivery, and policy each address essential aspects of the challenge, but often without shared planning frameworks or coordinated implementation. As a result, even well-designed and well-funded efforts can struggle to scale, align, or endure.

I did not arrive at this perspective from a single role or institution. I arrived at it by listening—across states, sectors, and systems. As a bedside nurse, public health leader, education policy fellow, nonprofit founder, and statewide nursing association president, I repeatedly encountered the same pattern: talented individuals navigating pathways that were more complex and disconnected than they needed to be. Students were eager but underprepared. Faculty were committed but stretched beyond capacity. Employers needed nurses while facing constraints on how training could expand. Many programs operate effectively within their own mandates, yet lack formal pathways for coordination across systems.

The recurring challenge was not a lack of solutions or investment, but the absence of coordination across systems.

This book does not claim to invent ideas in isolation. Instead, it intentionally integrates decades of workforce research, international policy guidance, and community-based practice to illuminate how these systems interact, where alignment breaks down, and why piece-meal solutions persist. My contribution is the design of an original framework that translates fragmented evidence, lived experience, and policy into a coherent, actionable strategy for leaders.

The NEXUS Nursing Framework is offered as that organizing lens. It identifies five interdependent elements—education, capacity, mobility, universal digital access, and structural equity—that together shape the nursing workforce. These elements already exist in practice, but they are rarely aligned intentionally. Naming them allows stakeholders across sectors to see the full system, understand their interdependence, and act with intention rather than urgency alone.

This book is written for policymakers, educators, health system leaders, workforce professionals, and nurses themselves—anyone invested in the future of nursing and the health of the communities it serves. It is both diagnostic and practical. It asks readers to build on the substantial work already underway while moving toward shared responsibility for strengthening the infrastructure that nursing depends on.

The nursing workforce should not be viewed solely as a staffing problem.

It should be understood as infrastructure.

And infrastructure is something we can choose to build—together.

# ACKNOWLEDGMENTS

This book emerged from a collective journey shaped by communities, colleagues, and institutions across multiple states that taught me valuable lessons about the realities of nursing workforce development. My understanding of nursing infrastructure began in Virginia, where I earned my nursing degree at Hampton University, a historically Black institution that demonstrated how intentional support transforms aspiring students into exceptional nurses. Hampton taught me that pathways to nursing are never neutral—they either remove barriers or reinforce them.

To the Virginia nursing community, including my colleagues at the Virginia Nurses Association, thank you for the opportunity to serve and for the work we shared to advance nursing across the state.

My early workforce development experience in New Jersey, particularly through the WorkFirst NJ initiative, taught me how workforce policy either enables or blocks access to career pathways. To the families, case managers, and administrators I worked alongside: you reminded me that "workforce development" is not an abstract concept—it includes economic survival, family stability, and community transformation.

My immersion in education policy as a DC Education Policy Fellow opened my eyes to how K–12, workforce development and higher education systems are structured in ways that can limit coordination around student success. That experience allowed me to see policy infrastructure not as it appears in agency reports, but as students experience it: disconnected, inconsistent, and often impossible to navigate. To the teachers—from elementary through high school—who introduce students to science, health careers, and the possibility of nursing: you are doing infrastructure work, even when the system does not name it as such. You are often the first—and sometimes the only—person who tells a student, "You could be a nurse." That matters more than policy can measure.

My foundational work in maternal and child health and public health grounded everything that followed. To the mothers, families, and children I served early in my career: you taught me that nursing is infrastructure. When that infrastructure falters, the ripple effects extend far beyond hospitals—into schools, homes, and entire communities.

To the nursing leaders who reviewed and endorsed this work and generously lent their credibility to its vision: Dr. Ernest Grant, Dr. Rebecca Patton, Mr. Sheldon Fields, and Dr. Olga Yakusheva—your willingness to champion this vision means everything.

To the Institute for Health and Social Equity (IHSE) community and the students we've supported through scholarship and mentorship: you are the reason this framework exists. Your persistence in the face of systemic barriers proves that talent is everywhere, although opportunity is not. You deserve infrastructure that matches your dedication.

To my parents, who taught me that education is both a personal right and a pathway to community transformation, thank you for your unwavering support and for showing me what dedication to serving others truly means.

Finally, to every nursing student who has been told there are no seats available, every CNA working nights while pursuing an RN, every LPN striving to advance in a system that was not designed to support seamless mobility, every high school counselor trying to navigate disconnected systems, every advisor stretching to help students find pathways that should not be this hard to find, and every faculty member serving more students than the system was designed to accommodate—this book is for you.

The nursing workforce should not be viewed as a staffing problem. It should be seen as infrastructure. And infrastructure is something we can—and must—rebuild together.

# PART I

# THE UNTOLD STORY OF THE NURSING WORKFORCE CRISIS

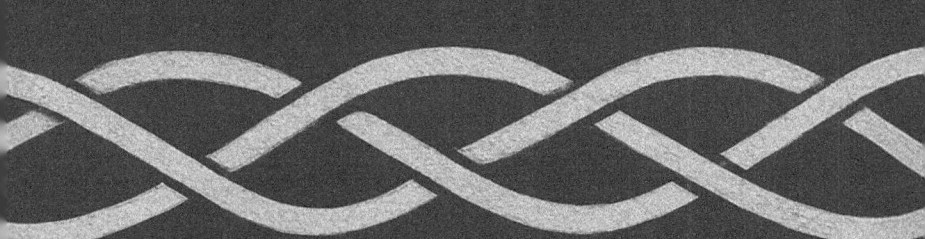

# The Nursing Workforce Crisis Is an Infrastructure Issue, Not a Shortage Problem

Most conversations about the nursing workforce focus on one familiar phrase: the nursing shortage. It has been the headline for decades, referring to a recurring crisis framed as a staffing problem for hospitals to solve or a recruitment problem for human resources departments to tackle.

## A GLOBAL INFRASTRUCTURE CHALLENGE

The nursing workforce crisis is not uniquely American. According to the World Health Organization (WHO, 2020), the world faces a projected shortage of 6 million nurses by 2030, with the most severe gaps in low- and middle-income countries. The Organisation for Economic Co-operation and Development (OECD, 2023) has documented similar patterns across member states: an aging workforce, capacity constraints in nursing education, insufficient clinical training infrastructure, and policy fragmentation that prevents coordinated workforce planning.

What we're experiencing in the United States mirrors the global pattern—nursing is essential infrastructure, yet it's treated as an afterthought in national planning. Countries that have made progress—such as those with integrated health workforce planning systems—demonstrate that outcomes improve dramatically when nursing is treated as infrastructure.

The distinction is clear: While other nations are beginning to align education, workforce development, and healthcare delivery systems, the United States continues to operate in silos. This book offers a framework designed to address and correct that problem.

## THE U.S. CONTEXT

*Stepping back reveals a broader reality.*

Nurses are not simply employees inside healthcare systems. We are the backbone of every community's well-being—across clinical care, economic stability, education, and public health. When the nursing workforce falters, ripple effects reach far beyond the hospital: schools lose support, public health systems strain, local employers struggle with absenteeism, maternal and child health outcomes worsen, and entire regions become medically fragile.

This is why we must shift the narrative:

> *The nursing workforce is not a staffing issue. The nursing workforce should be seen as infrastructure.*

Just like roads, broadband, clean water, and electricity, a functioning nursing workforce determines whether a society thrives or collapses. When nursing infrastructure is strong, communities experience stability, safety, continuity, and growth. When it breaks down, everything else begins to crumble.

### A NOTE ON LANGUAGE: *PATHWAY* VS. *PIPELINE*

Throughout this book, I use the term *pathway* rather than *pipeline* to describe pathways into nursing. This choice is intentional. The metaphor of a pipeline suggests a narrow, rigid pathway—one direction, one diameter, one flow. Nursing pathways are far more dynamic. They involve multiple entry points, varied speeds of progression, and opportunities to exit and reenter as life circumstances change.

Additionally, the term *pipeline* has become politically charged, particularly for Indigenous communities and those concerned with environmental justice. Language matters in policy work, and I choose terms that honor both the complexity of human pathways and the dignity of all communities.

### AN EXAMPLE FROM MY EARLY CAREER

Early in my public health career, I worked in a region where a single nurse's retirement revealed just how fragile maternal-child home visiting services really were. One departure—one gap in infrastructure—meant remaining staff absorbed crushing workloads to ensure no family was turned away. But something had to give. Visits became shorter and less frequent, and the depth of care families received—the extended postpartum monitoring, the thorough breastfeeding support, the comprehensive home-based assessment—was reduced to the bare minimum.

In another community, the loss of two school nurses meant hundreds of children with asthma, diabetes, seizures, and chronic conditions were left without consistent medical oversight for weeks. Teachers and counselors—committed professionals without medical training—found themselves making decisions about medication administration, emergency response, and health management that should never fall to education staff. When the infrastructure breaks down, everyone improvises. But improvisation in healthcare carries risk.

What I describe above were not staffing challenges but infrastructure failures, with consequences that touched education, health, safety, and family stability. Beyond hospitals and clinics, nurses serve in roles many people never see: parish nurses in faith communities providing health monitoring for elderly congregants, occupational health nurses in factories and agricultural settings managing workplace injuries, and public health nurses conducting maternal-child home visits. Each of these roles represents essential infrastructure. When a parish nurse retires from a faith community, that community loses its primary health monitoring system. When an occupational health nurse position goes unfilled at a manufacturing plant, workplace injuries go unaddressed and productivity drops. These are not isolated staffing problems—they are infrastructure gaps with cascading effects across entire communities.

However, nursing's infrastructure role extends far beyond hospitals and clinics. When the nursing workforce destabilizes, the effects ripple across the entire economy in ways most people never see coming.

Consider what happens when surgical suites can't open because there aren't enough perioperative nurses. Elective procedures get postponed—sometimes for months. Medical device manufacturers see revenue drop. Surgical supply chains adjust production schedules. Insurance companies restructure risk models as preventable conditions worsen without intervention. The finance sector tracks these workforce gaps as economic indicators.

Or think about transportation. Every commercial truck driver, airline pilot, and transit worker needs regular health screenings and Department of Transportation physicals. When occupational health nurses aren't available, drivers sit idle. Goods don't move, and supply chains break. The same pattern plays out in manufacturing—workplace injuries go unaddressed without occupational health nurses, which leads to lost productivity, increased workers' compensation claims, and reduced output.

In agricultural communities, especially those supporting migrant and seasonal workers, access to primary care often depends on a single rural health clinic staffed by nurse practitioners. When that position goes unfilled, entire communities lose access to healthcare. Crop yields can suffer when workers can't access treatment for heat-related illness or occupational injuries. And this is how food security becomes a workforce issue.

Energy sector workers in remote locations (e.g., offshore platforms, pipeline stations, and wind farms) depend on telemedicine and emergency response systems staffed by nurses. Technology companies building AI-powered health tools need nurses to design, test, and implement them. Schools can't function safely without school nurses managing chronic conditions, administering medications, and responding to emergencies. Even national security depends on military readiness, which requires healthcare workforce capacity to support service members, veterans, and their families.

The coronavirus (COVID-19) pandemic made these dependencies visible in ways they'd never been before. When intensive care units filled and nurses burned out, elective surgeries stopped nationwide. Cancer screenings were delayed. Routine preventive care vanished. The economic consequences were swift and severe—not just for hospitals, but for medical supply companies, insurance carriers, pharmaceutical distributors, and every sector that depends on a healthy, productive workforce.

Climate change is intensifying these dependencies. Extreme weather events—hurricanes, wildfires, floods, heat waves—require rapid healthcare surge capacity. Nurses staff emergency shelters, coordinate disaster response, and provide care in mobile clinics. As climate-related health impacts grow, so does the need for nursing workforce resilience. This isn't a healthcare issue—it's an infrastructure issue affecting disaster preparedness, community resilience, and national security.

That's why The NEXUS Nursing Framework™ positions nursing workforce development as essential infrastructure, not isolated healthcare planning.

When finance, manufacturing, transportation, agriculture, energy, technology, education, housing, food systems, climate response, and national defense all depend on nursing workforce stability, the conversation can't stay siloed within healthcare. Governors, economic development officials, workforce boards, and business leaders need to understand that investing in nursing infrastructure isn't just about hospitals but about economic stability and national resilience.

## WHAT CHANGES WHEN WE REFRAME THIS

When we frame nursing as infrastructure, everything changes:

- We stop treating shortages as temporary crises.

- We stop relying solely on hospitals to fix a national issue.

- We start looking at the entire education-to-workforce pathway.

- We begin recognizing the interconnected systems that shape entry, mobility, and retention.

This leads to a more urgent question:

> *If nursing is infrastructure, why is the system that produces nurses so misaligned?*

To answer, we turn to real stories of what aspiring nurses are experiencing long before they ever apply to nursing school. The NEXUS Nursing Framework is intended to complement and strengthen the extensive work already underway across nursing organizations, academic institutions, and policy bodies—not replace it.

# CHAPTER 2

# Why Our Current System Fails

## *A Real Story From the Field*

Let's begin with a story that illustrates how infrastructure gaps affect real people navigating these systems.

A few years ago, at a high school where students were passionate about becoming nurses, their teacher—full of enthusiasm and dedication—did everything she could with what she had.

But their lab was a storage closet.

One outdated hospital bed was wedged between boxes of cleaning supplies. There were no gloves, no mannequins, no monitors, no simulation tools. The teacher wasn't certified to teach health science. There were no dual enrollment options. No nursing pathways. No clinical exposure. No advisory partnerships.

And yet these students came from a community with some of the greatest need for nurses.

This is what policy misalignment looks like in real life.

## ANOTHER STORY:
## WHEN SYSTEMS DON'T TALK

Throughout my workforce development career, I've encountered the following pattern: Workforce counselors say, "My clients want to pursue nursing, but they need science prerequisites first, and our funding won't cover college courses."

College advisors say, "We have seats open in our prerequisite courses, but adult students don't qualify for financial aid until there's a degree program."

Both are right. Both are frustrated. The gap between workforce funding and education funding keeps qualified adults from ever starting.

That is not a people problem. That is a systems problem.

## FINDING THE MISALIGNMENT

Federal and state data confirm what these stories illustrate: access to foundational preparation varies dramatically by geography, race, and income.

Many schools—especially those in rural, underfunded, and historically marginalized communities—lack

- Updated science laboratories

- Certified health science teachers

- Dual-enrollment opportunities

- Meaningful career advising

- Work-based learning experiences

- Industry partnerships

So when policymakers ask why the nursing workforce isn't diverse, practice-ready, or large enough—these are the reasons why.

However, the misalignment doesn't stop there.

## THE NEXT BARRIER: HIGHER EDUCATION CAPACITY

Even when students manage to reach college, they run into

- Faculty shortages

- Limited clinical placements

- Uneven simulation access

- Budget constraints

- Long waiting lists

These capacity barriers mean qualified students are turned away every year—not because they aren't ready, but because the system isn't ready.

## THE ADULT LEARNER BARRIER: THE WIOA GAP

And for adult learners—working parents, career changers, returning students—the Workforce Innovation and Opportunity Act (WIOA) poses another challenge. WIOA is the nation's primary federal law that funds job training and workforce development programs provided through state and local workforce boards. It was designed to support rapid employment through short-term training programs, typically 6–12 weeks. However, nursing education requires multiyear clinical training; prerequisites in anatomy, physiology, and microbiology; and extensive supervised practice. This fundamental mismatch creates a critical gap in workforce funding.

The above-mentioned means that adult learners who want to become nurses are often stranded by

- Too few financial supports

- Too many competing responsibilities

- Not enough flexible pathways

## THE BOTTOM LINE

The system isn't broken because people don't care. It's broken because the policies that shape nursing preparation were never designed to work together.

The NEXUS Nursing Framework is one response to this challenge, offering a policy-aligned approach to addressing these structural gaps.

# CHAPTER 3

# The NEXUS Nursing Framework™

*A Simple Way to*
*Understand a Complex System*

M ost people, including those in education or healthcare, interact only with one part of the nursing workforce ecosystem.

A nurse educator may understand Title VIII. A workforce leader may understand WIOA. A high school CTE director may understand Perkins V. A hospital executive may understand reimbursement models and staffing ratios—but not the education pathway that produces the nurses they need.

Very few see all five elements that determine whether someone can become a nurse—and whether nurses stay in the profession once they're there. Infrastructure failures don't just block entry; they drive experienced nurses out. Faculty shortages create unsustainable workloads. Digital systems consume hours that should go to patient care.

Lack of advancement pathways sends talented CNAs and LPNs out of healthcare entirely.

This isn't a knowledge gap but a system design gap.

## A GROUNDING INSIGHT
## FROM MY INTERVIEWS

In one interview, a workforce board leader said, "We can support CNA and CMA training, but we can't fund 2-year degrees."

A week later, a nursing dean told me, "We have a full faculty ready to teach, but the clinical site withdrew last minute."

Both leaders were right. Neither one had full context. Both were operating inside separate federal frameworks with no shared alignment.

## THE GLOBAL CONTEXT:
## MINISTRY SILOS ARE UNIVERSAL

The challenge of fragmented workforce systems is not unique to the United States. OECD research on workforce development has consistently identified "ministry silos" as a primary barrier to effective health workforce planning (OECD, 2019). In most countries, education and health ministries, labor departments, and finance agencies operate independently, creating the exact misalignments we see domestically.

Nations that have successfully addressed nursing shortages—such as Australia's coordinated Health Workforce Australia initiative or the United Kingdom's NHS Long Term Workforce Plan—did so by creating cross-sector coordination mechanisms that bridge these gaps (Health Workforce Australia, 2014; NHS England, 2023; OECD, 2023). The NEXUS Framework offers a similar approach in the United States, adapted to the federal system and state-level implementation realities.

# THE NEXUS NURSING FRAMEWORK™

The NEXUS Framework organizes the fragmentation into five elements that shape the nursing workforce:

## N–Nursing Education Infrastructure

*K–12 exposure + early academic preparation*

Includes health science pathways, dual enrollment, labs, advising, and CTE programs

Fragmented K–12 preparation → Fewer prepared nursing students

## E–Educational Capacity

*The ability of higher education institutions to train nurses*

Involves faculty availability, clinical placements, simulation resources, and technological capacity

Capacity limits → Qualified students turned away

## X–Cross-sector Mobility

*Adult entry + advancement pathways*

Includes apprenticeships, stackable credentials, WIOA funding, supportive services, and flexible schedules

Misaligned systems → Adults are unable to enter or advance

## U–Universal Digital Access

*Simulation, AI, informatics, telehealth, broadband*

The future of nursing is digital, but access is deeply unequal.

Digital divide → Uneven readiness for modern practice

## S–Structural Equity

*Equity at every stage*

Race, income, geography, systemic barriers, historic disinvestment

## EQUITY GAPS → REPEATED
## DISADVANTAGE ACROSS GENERATIONS

Once the elements are visible together, patterns that once felt disconnected begin to make sense:

- Shortages become understandable.

- Breakdowns are easier to identify.

- Policy solutions become actionable.

- Educators, employers, and policymakers can speak a common language.

That is the power of the NEXUS Nursing Framework™.

*Figure 3.1 on the next page illustrates how misaligned federal policies create gaps across the nursing education-to-workforce pathway.*

Three major federal funding streams—Perkins V, WIOA, and Title VIII—operate independently, creating critical gaps across the nursing education-to-workforce pathway. The NEXUS Nursing Framework proposes braiding these policies to support a continuous student journey.

*Instructors, policymakers, and institutional partners may access a full-color reference version of this original visual at: nexusnursingframework.com*

# FEDERAL POLICY GAPS IN THE NURSING WORKFORCE SYSTEM

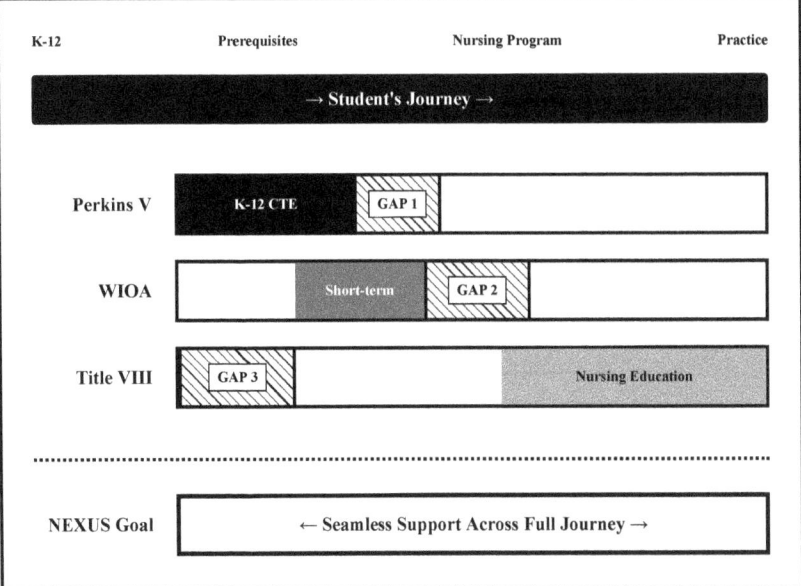

## THREE CRITICAL POLICY GAPS

### Perkins V → WIOA: "Aging Out"

High school health pathway graduates lose structured support when transitioning to adult workforce programs. 18-20 year olds fall through while completing prerequisites.

### WIOA → Title VIII: "Too Long"

WIOA's structure prioritizes short-term training, which may not align with the sequencing of nursing education, resulting in interruptions to workforce-funded supports for adult learners during preparation phases.

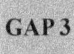

### Perkins V → Title VIII: "Coordination"

Systematic coordination between K-12 health pathways and nursing programs is not universal. Students experience inconsistent academic preparation and credit transfer policies, requiring many to repeat coursework or remediate gaps.

---

### THE NEXUS FRAMEWORK™ SOLUTION

**Braid** Perkins V, WIOA, and Title VIII around the student journey to close all three gaps.

---

FIGURE 3.1. Source: *The NEXUS Nursing Framework™.* © 2025 Dr. Sherri Johnson.

# CHAPTER 4

# What K–12 Educators See That Policymakers Miss

I f we're honest, most conversations about the nursing workforce skip right over the people who see talent first: K–12 teachers. Not nursing faculty, not hospital executives, not policymakers but teachers.

Elementary teachers see the student who lights up during science lessons. Middle school teachers see the student who instinctively wants to help a classmate who's hurt. High school CTE teachers see the student who stays after school to practice taking vitals or wants to shadow a nurse at a local clinic.

Teachers see leadership and compassion before any standardized test, college acceptance, or NCLEX exam ever enters the picture.

So, if we truly want to fix the nursing pathway, we cannot begin at community college. We cannot begin at the BSN program. We cannot even begin at age 16.

We have to begin much earlier. And that's where our policies fall apart.

## A GLOBAL PATTERN:
## EARLY PATHWAYS MATTER

Research from the OECD and World Bank consistently shows that countries with strong K–12 career pathway systems—particularly in vocational and technical education—produce more qualified applicants for healthcare professions (OECD, 2020; World Bank, 2018). Nations such as Germany, Switzerland, and Singapore integrate career exposure and skill-building into secondary education, creating smoother transitions into healthcare training.

By contrast, the United States has largely separated career and technical education from college preparation, which creates artificial barriers that other nations have successfully avoided. When the World Economic Forum (2020) analyzed health workforce competitiveness, early career pathway access consistently emerged as a differentiator between high-performing and struggling systems.

## A COMPOSITE STORY FROM
## CLASSROOMS ACROSS THE COUNTRY

In communities across the United States, I've heard the same pattern from teachers and youth leaders. They describe students who are compassionate, curious, and naturally drawn to helping others—young people who would thrive in nursing, STEM, or public health careers.

And yet, because of how unaligned our national education and workforce systems are, many students move through middle school and even into high school with little or no exposure to these fields.

There are no structured opportunities to explore health or science careers and no mentorship from professionals in the field. The access to hands-on labs or equipment is limited, and there are few programs that help students understand what these careers look like in real life. And this is so not because educators don't care but because the system doesn't give them the resources or support.

These are the early losses we rarely talk about: The young people who might have become nurses, scientists, or public health leaders if they had known the path existed.

This is part of why I founded the Institute for Health and Social Equity (IHSE) years ago—to provide scholarships, mentoring, and exposure for students who might otherwise be overlooked. Our work has shown me repeatedly how powerful early guidance and access can be. When students see what's possible, everything changes.

## THE K-12 REALITY THAT POLICYMAKERS RARELY SEE

The patterns I describe here are not tied to any single system, program, or employer. They reflect what I've learned across years of working at the intersections of *nursing, public health, community partnerships, and education policy*—including my time as an *Education Policy Fellow* and my work through the IHSE.

Across communities nationwide, teachers and youth leaders describe the same challenges:

### 1. Uneven Access to Foundational Science

In many schools—especially those serving under-resourced communities—students do not consistently have access to adequate lab equipment, updated science materials, inquiry-based curriculum, or qualified science or CTE teachers.

These gaps don't reflect a lack of student talent but a lack of opportunity.

### 2. Guidance Counselors Stretched Beyond Capacity

In many schools, one counselor supports 300–500 students, sometimes even more. Career exploration becomes reactive instead of strategic.

Consequently, students who might thrive in health careers may not receive meaningful exposure until it's too late to choose the courses that prepare them.

### 3. Limited Dual Enrollment or Health Science Pathways

This remains particularly common in rural communities, underfunded school systems, and under-resourced urban communities.

Many students graduate without ever taking anatomy, medical terminology, biology labs, health science electives, or introductory courses such as phlebotomy or patient care fundamentals.

You cannot pursue what you cannot see.

### 4. Teachers as De Facto Career Advisors

Teachers often serve as mentors, career coaches, advocates, and connectors to opportunities—all on top of their full instructional load.

Too often, the extent to which the future workforce depends on this unpaid and largely invisible labor is built into systems without being formally acknowledged or supported.

## THE NEXUS NURSING FRAMEWORK™ APPLIED TO K–12

Let's apply The NEXUS Nursing Framework to the perspective of a teacher, principal, or superintendent.

### N–Nursing Education Infrastructure

K–12 is the birthplace of the nursing workforce. This includes

STEM readiness, reading and writing skills, early exposure to science, health pathways, and school culture around leadership and service.

When these elements are underdeveloped or uneven, the nursing pathway often narrows long before it begins.

### E—*Educational Capacity (But for K–12)*

Educational capacity isn't just a college issue. K–12 teacher shortages—especially in science, math, and health-related fields—directly constrain the nursing workforce pathway.

To illustrate this downstream effect: if a school system cannot hire a single biology teacher, this can represent approximately six potential nurses lost over the course of that teacher's tenure (see Appendix F for calculation methodology used throughout this book).

### X—*Cross-Sector Mobility for Students*

This is where equity becomes visible. Students need reliable transportation, access to summer programs, support for internships, and opportunities to visit colleges and hospitals.

Without mobility supports, students in rural and resource-limited communities face barriers before they even get started.

Without mobility, students in rural and resource-limited communities fall behind before they even get started.

### U—*Universal Digital Access*

Not every student has access to devices, broadband, virtual labs, simulation tools, or online dual enrollment.

Digital divides in middle school often become readiness divides in college.

### S—Structural Equity

Students who are first-generation, live in low-income households, attend underfunded schools, or have fewer community resources encounter structural barriers long before nursing school applications.

Teachers see this every day.

## A TEACHER'S PERSPECTIVE ON "THE NURSING SHORTAGE"

I once asked a group of high school teachers, "When you hear 'nursing shortage,' what comes to mind?"

Their answers were telling:

- "We don't have the equipment to prepare students."

- "Students can't take the right classes."

- "Parents don't understand the pathway."

- "Our kids want to be nurses, but colleges keep turning them away."

- "We need partnerships—but we don't have capacity to set them up."

Every single answer came from *inside* their school buildings—not hospitals or universities.

We cannot solve the nursing crisis without listening to K–12 educators.

## POLICY TAKEAWAY

If the goal is to increase the nursing workforce, we must treat K–12 as a fully integrated part of the nursing pathway, not an optional "early exposure" phase.

This means

- Health science pathways in every high school

- STEM foundations beginning in elementary school

- Dual enrollment aligned with nursing programs

- CTE teachers supported and certified

- Funding for labs and career counseling

- Partnerships between schools and health systems

- Regional career hubs

- Transportation for internships and pathways

- Parent and community engagement

Teachers cannot shoulder this alone. States, systems, and policymakers must build infrastructure that connects K–12 to the rest of the pathway intentionally.

# CHAPTER 5

# The Power of Community

*What Scholarships, Mentors, and Belief Can Build*

Before I became a nurse, a policy strategist, and the founder of an equity-focused institute, I was a student who needed more than visibility—I needed someone to understand my learning needs and meet me where I was. That experience shaped how I show up for young people today: with empathy, patience, and a commitment to seeing not just who they are, but what they need to thrive.

## COMMUNITY-BASED SUPPORT: A GLOBAL BEST PRACTICE

Community-based scholarship and mentorship programs are recognized globally as essential infrastructure for health workforce development. Research from the World Bank's Human Capital Project demonstrates that countries achieving equitable healthcare workforce distribution consistently invest in community-level support systems—particularly for students from underrepresented regions (World Bank, 2023).

Organizations like IHSE represent the kind of grassroots infrastructure that complements formal education systems. While other nations embed these supports into national policy frameworks, the United States relies heavily on nonprofit and community-driven initiatives to fill systemic gaps.

Every chapter in this book, the framework I developed, and every recommendation I offer draws from both policy analysis and lived experience. That is because long before I wrote about systems, I lived inside them.

I've seen firsthand what happens when the right support shows up at the right time. Not just in my own life, but in the lives of countless young people I've encountered through IHSE. When students receive individualized guidance, affirmation, and access, their entire trajectory can shift.

This chapter is about that kind of support—the support that changes pathways long before a student ever steps into a nursing program.

## A PERSONAL STORY:
## BUILDING THE BRIDGE I NEEDED

I didn't grow up in a formalized academic pathway aligned to health careers, but I also wasn't without guidance. By high school, I knew I wanted to be a nurse. That clarity emerged through intentional exposure—participating in an early program called *Medical Explorers*, volunteering at our local hospital, and completing rotations that allowed me to shadow operating room nurses and see the profession up close.

My parents understood what I needed even when the school system didn't offer it. They stewarded my dream—seeking out enrichment opportunities, supporting my volunteer work, and ensuring I had the exposure that confirmed my calling. *Medical Explorers* wasn't just a spark; it was validation of what I already felt pulled toward.

What I didn't have was a coordinated, system-supported pathway designed to carry students from early interest into nursing education. I didn't have a full scholarship package waiting for me. I didn't have a seamless structure connecting my high school experiences to college nursing programs. The bridge-building fell to my family—and to me.

There were moments when tuition was a struggle and when books were too expensive. Moments when I had to choose between work hours and clinical hours. Moments when I felt out of place in rooms that didn't always feel built for me.

And still—I kept going.

Not because I was figuring it out alone, but because my parents gave me something essential: the belief that my dream was legitimate and the support to pursue it, even when the system made the journey harder than it needed to be.

What I didn't have was an organization like IHSE walking alongside students the way we do today.

That's why I know what it feels like to need a bridge—and exactly what it costs when one isn't there.

## IHSE: WHERE EQUITY BECOMES ACTION

Running IHSE has given me a front-row seat to the ways small interventions can create generational change.

We've supported students who

- Are first in their family to graduate
- Come from rural communities with limited opportunities
- Attend schools without health science pathways
- Navigate caregiving responsibilities at home
- Balance work and study
- Experience hardship and still rise

Our scholarships are not large—and yet, they are transformative. We've seen $500 change a student's semester. We've seen $1,000 keep a student enrolled. We've seen $1,500 cover exam fees, uniforms, transportation, or housing gaps—the very things policymakers forget when designing systems.

And we've seen something else too: When a young person knows someone believes in them, they walk differently.

Scholarship dollars matter—but belief capital matters too.

You can see it in their eyes. You can hear it in their voice. You can feel it in their posture.

Confidence is its own kind of currency.

## WHAT SCHOLARSHIPS REVEAL ABOUT THE TALENT STREAM

Here's what IHSE has taught me about the nursing and STEM pathway:

### 1. Talent is universal. Opportunity is not.

We have brilliant students everywhere—rural, urban, suburban, wealthy, low-income. The difference is not in their potential. The difference is exposure, resources, and belief.

### 2. Most students don't fail academically—they fail logistically.

They have to deal with financial stress, transportation., childcare, books, lab fees, uniforms, technology, housing insecurity, and the cost of just "being a student."

These are system failures, not student failures.

### 3. Small investments create disproportionate impact.

A $250 test fee can determine whether a student becomes a nurse. A $75 uniform can determine whether a student stays in clinicals. A bus pass can determine whether a student finishes the semester.

We don't talk about these things in policy discussions—but they are the real-world barriers that shape the workforce.

### 4. Community matters as much as curriculum.

Students thrive in supportive ecosystems: mentors, caring teachers, access to networks, spiritual grounding, financial support, and clear pathways.

This is the "equity infrastructure" my framework refers to—and IHSE has proven it works.

## A K-12 SCHOLARSHIP STORY: THE TWELFTH GRADER WHO BECAME A NURSE

One year, IHSE awarded a scholarship to a 12th grade student from a rural school. She didn't have a pathway at her high school. No lab. No exposure. But she had a dream—she wanted to be a nurse.

Our scholarship wasn't about tuition. It funded

- Transportation support
- Essential Supplies
- Access to volunteer mentorship and guided exposure opportunities

She is now a Registered Nurse serving a rural population. She wrote to us recently:

> *"You saw me before anyone else did. Thank you for helping me become what I always knew I could be."*

This is why K–12 matters. This is why scholarships matter. This is why The NEXUS Nursing Framework begins long before college.

## POLICY LESSON: SCHOLARSHIPS ARE INFRASTRUCTURE

In The NEXUS Nursing Framework, we talk about "structural equity." But that language can feel abstract. Here's a translation:

> *A scholarship is infrastructure. A bus pass is infrastructure. A mentor is infrastructure. A dual enrollment opportunity is infrastructure. A supportive teacher is infrastructure. A school counselor who actually has time is infrastructure. A summer program is infrastructure. A caring community is infrastructure.*

These are the things that remove friction from a student's path.

When policymakers ask, "How do we fix the nursing shortage?" this is one of the answers.

We must engineer environments of support, not just environments of instruction.

## A PERSONAL REFLECTION

This part of the work has always felt meaningful to me in a way that goes beyond policy. When you invest in a young person's future—especially someone who has been overlooked—you're participating in their becoming. You're offering support at a moment when it can shift a trajectory.

Very often, the right people appear at the right time—teachers, mentors, donors, community leaders, and advocates.

I've been on the receiving end of that kind of timely support. And through IHSE, I now have the privilege of helping to extend it to others.

## WHERE WE GO FROM HERE

This chapter represents the heart beneath the policy. The human side. It is the side that is often overlooked by decision-makers, carried daily by teachers, and known instinctively by nurses—the side that defines why this work matters.

If we want to build a future-ready nursing workforce—one that is diverse, ethical, steadfast, and prepared—we have to invest in

- K–12 teachers
- Families
- Communities
- Faith-based partners

- Financial support systems

- Early exposure programs

- Leadership development

- Pathways that start well before senior year

When we do that, we don't just produce nurses. We produce leaders. We produce purpose-driven professionals. We produce changemakers. We produce the workforce our communities deserve.

# CHAPTER 6

# What Nurses See

*The Reality From the Bedside*
*That Policy Can't Ignore*

I f you want to understand the nursing workforce, you cannot start with a spreadsheet. You cannot start with a policy memo. You cannot start with an economic forecast, a workforce report, or a legislative hearing.

You must start where the story actually lives at the bedside.

## THE GLOBAL NURSING VOICE

Across nations, nurses report strikingly similar experiences: moral distress from inadequate staffing, frustration with fragmented systems, and the burden of being society's most trusted professionals yet least heard voices in policy. The International Council of Nurses (ICN, 2021) and WHO's State of the World's Nursing reports consistently document these patterns.

What distinguishes the United States is not the nature of these challenges, but our failure to systematically include nurses in workforce planning. Countries with effective health workforce strategies—from Scandinavia to New Zealand—place nurses at the center of policy design, not at the margins (WHO, 2022).

This is because nurses see things nobody else sees—not administrators, not policymakers, not even the data analysts who study the workforce.

Nurses see society. Nurses see systems. Nurses see inequity in real time. They see trauma, courage, and failure up close. Nurses see what works and what absolutely does not.

And because nurses are everywhere—schools, public health departments, community clinics, hospitals, telehealth, correctional facilities, home care—they have a view of the world that is more comprehensive than any single sector.

We see it all.

Throughout my years in nursing leadership, I witnessed stories from every corner of the profession. Stories that were heartbreaking, hopeful, energizing, frustrating, and prophetic. Stories that never make it into policy briefs. Stories that become the "real data" behind The NEXUS Nursing Framework

This chapter is about those stories—the ones nurses carry quietly until someone finally asks.

## WHEN ONE NURSE SPEAKS FOR THOUSANDS

One nurse told me, with tears in her eyes:

> *"I am burnt out and distressed. I know what my patients deserve, but I can't give it to them with what we have."*

This wasn't a shortage of compassion. It was a shortage of infrastructure. What that nurse was describing was:

- Moral distress
- Burnout
- Understaffing
- Lack of supplies
- Excessive patient loads
- Broken communication systems
- Outdated equipment
- Fatigued teams
- Unsafe ratios
- Unrealistic expectations

This was system failure showing up in one person's body.

Even as awareness of workplace environment and wellness has grown, system-level responses to burnout have often centered on short-term, symptom-focused interventions rather than structural change.

But nurses experience the consequences of those choices differently:

- *Be stronger with fewer resources.*
- *Do more with less.*
- *Carry the weight of structural failures quietly.*

The NEXUS Nursing Framework tells us this clearly: shortages are not about people—they're about systems.

The bedside nurses know this. They feel it in their bones.

## SECTION 1: PUBLIC HEALTH NURSES

*A story from a public health nurse who saw the crisis before the headlines*

In my years working as a public health nurse, I lived this reality—and heard it echoed in conversations with colleagues across the field. We were the ones monitoring trends long before the rest of the world noticed something was wrong.

One colleague once captured it perfectly:

> *"By the time the public sees the problem, we've been seeing it for months."*

Public health nurses are often the earliest warning system for our communities. We see

- Rising chronic disease rates

- Maternal health inequities

- Infectious disease patterns

- Mental health concerns

- Community violence as a public health issue

But here's the truth: public health nurses are often compensated at lower levels than acute care nurses, are understaffed and underfunded, are expected to cover large geographic areas, and are not routinely included in cross-sector workforce and infrastructure conversations.

This is exactly why structural alignment matters so much. We have a system where the professionals with the clearest, earliest information often have the fewest resources to act on it.

Imagine if public health nurses were consistently centered in strategy and funding decisions—not only within health departments, but alongside sectors such as finance, transportation, housing, and education as part of broader infrastructure planning and investment. In places where this approach has been piloted, it has supported earlier intervention and informed strategies to reduce downstream crises. Scaling that model would allow us to prevent emergencies rather than simply react to them.

## SECTION 2: SCHOOL NURSES

### What School Nurses See Every Day

When we talk about the education-to-career landscape, we cannot overlook school nurses. For many children, the school nurse is the only health professional they will consistently encounter.

A school nurse once shared with me:

> *"I'm the counselor, the triage nurse, the social worker, the parent whisperer, and the public health department—all in one."*

And she wasn't exaggerating.

In some communities, one nurse covers two or three schools. In others, there's no school nurse at all.

They see

- Unmanaged asthma

- Food insecurity

- Mental health crises

- Chronic illness with no primary care support

- Students caring for younger siblings

- Students working full time after school

- Instability at home

- Violence

- Homelessness

- Child abuse

When a student faints in class, it's not always dehydration. Sometimes it's hunger. Sometimes it's trauma. Sometimes it's the weight of stress no one else saw.

And yet these same students are expected to pass biology, explore careers, and graduate prepared for what comes next.

We cannot talk about the future nursing workforce—or *any* workforce—without acknowledging the conditions children grow up in.

School nurses know this. Teachers know this. Communities know this. But policy almost never accounts for it.


## SECTION 3: NURSES ACROSS THE STATE

### *When Trust Doesn't Translate to Influence*

Nurses remain the most trusted profession in America—patients depend on us, families confide in us. Communities rely on our judgment in moments that matter most.

And yet, as I traveled statewide listening to nurses across all settings, I heard a consistent concern—not about trust, but about influence. Nurses spoke less about whether their voices were respected, and more about whether their expertise was meaningfully shaping the systems they work within.

The themes I heard repeatedly:

- "We offer solutions, people listen—and then the system stays the same."

- "If you want to know what's really happening, ask the nurse. If you want solutions that work, include the nurse."

- "We're exhausted, not defeated. We just need the systems we work in to be designed with our expertise, not despite it."

Across emergency rooms, long-term care, school health, public health, rural clinics, and academic settings, the message was consistent. The issue has never been a lack of:

- Dedication

- Talent

- Calling

The challenge is structural:

- Systems that are not fully aligned

- Decision-making processes that underutilize nursing expertise

- Workforce strategies developed *around* nurses rather than *with* them

And this is exactly where The NEXUS Nursing Framework comes in. It names what nurses have been saying for decades: we cannot solve a workforce crisis with isolated solutions. Sustainable progress requires alignment, coordination, and systems intentionally designed around the realities nurses see every day.

## A STORY THAT SHOWS
## WHY POLICY MUST CHANGE

During one legislative session, I was meeting with lawmakers to advocate for safer workplace conditions for nurses. In the middle of that hectic week, a nurse pulled me aside—exhausted after three back-to-back 12-hour shifts—and asked me to share her story with policymakers.

She didn't come to the Capitol because she had time. She reached out because she had courage. With tears running down her face, she said to me:

> *"If they fix the system, we can save more lives. Please don't make us choose between our safety and our calling."*

I carried her words into every conversation that day.

And I will never forget that moment—not because the information was new, but because the emotion behind it was undeniable.

Sometimes the system needs to hear the truth from the people living it, even when they can't be in the room themselves.

## POLICY LESSON: NURSES ARE
## THE SYSTEM'S TRUTH TELLERS

When nurses describe workforce challenges, they're not complaining—they're diagnosing. Nurses are the clinicians who:

- Document what's happening

- Assess the reality

- Identify patterns

- Anticipate deterioration

- Escalate concerns

- Recommend action steps

This is exactly the kind of thinking policymakers need.

Nurses don't just see patients—nurses see systems.

When a nurse says, "We need more staff," they're describing a capacity failure. When a nurse says, "We're losing new graduates," they're describing an education-to-practice alignment failure. When a nurse says, "Our community is struggling," they're describing an equity infrastructure failure.

This is why nurses must be at the center of workforce policy design—not at the margins.

## BRINGING IT ALL TOGETHER

K–12 educators see the potential. Public health nurses see the community. School nurses see the early signs. Clinical nurses see the consequences. Nurse leaders see the patterns. Policymakers see the budget.

But nurses—especially frontline nurses—hold the threads that connect all of these pieces.

In The NEXUS Nursing Framework, the "S" for Structural Equity and the "X" for Cross-sector Mobility depend on what nurses see every day.

Nursing doesn't operate in isolation. It lives in schools, community centers, emergency rooms, maternal health programs, long-term care facilities, public health clinics, and crisis units.

Nurses see the system in full view.

And until policymakers see through nurses' eyes, we will keep trying to fix symptoms instead of causes.

# CHAPTER 7

# Higher Education and Clinical Capacity

## *What Colleges and Clinical Partners Wish Policymakers Understood*

M ost people believe that if we simply "get more students interested in nursing," the workforce will fix itself. But people who work inside nursing schools—faculty, program directors, clinical coordinators, and deans—know the truth:

*Interest is not the problem. Capacity is.*

Every year across the country, thousands of students are turned away from nursing programs. Not because they lack potential, passion, or purpose but because the system can't hold them.

In my advocacy work, this was the issue that came up in nearly every meeting, every town hall, every legislative briefing, and every campus visit:

*"We have the students. We don't have the faculty, the clinical slots, or the resources."*

This isn't about a lack of willingness. It's about structural limits.

In The NEXUS Nursing Framework this is the **E: Education Educational Capacity**—the bottleneck that quietly caps the entire nation's workforce.

Let's look at what this means on the ground.

## CAPACITY CONSTRAINTS: A UNIVERSAL CHALLENGE

Nursing faculty shortages and clinical placement bottlenecks are global phenomena. The OECD's Health Workforce Migration report documents these constraints across member nations, noting that countries with aging nurse educator populations face particularly acute challenges (OECD, 2019). Australia, Canada, and the United Kingdom all report similar patterns: qualified applicants turned away due to limited clinical training sites and insufficient faculty.

What sets the United States apart is the fragmentation of solutions. While other nations coordinate faculty development, clinical site expansion, and simulation investment through centralized planning, U.S. nursing schools compete for resources within fragmented funding systems, which creates inefficiencies.

## A STORY FROM A COMMUNITY COLLEGE NURSING DEAN

During my work with nursing leaders across the state, a community college dean once shared something with me that I have never forgotten. As we discussed her program's enrollment challenges, she gestured toward a classroom of eager pre-nursing students and said:

*"If I had one additional faculty member, I could take* at *least thirty more students right now. I have qualified appli-cants. I have people waiting. What I don't have is another faculty member—or a clinical site."*

She then explained that many applicants had

- met the GPA requirement,
- completed all prerequisites,
- passed entrance exams,
- submitted thoughtful essays, and
- interviewed strongly

and still received a denial—not because they were unprepared, but because the system could not accommodate them.

This is the capacity crisis—and it begins long before a student ever reaches a hospital floor.

## THE FACULTY SHORTAGE: A CRISIS HIDDEN IN PLAIN SIGHT

Nursing faculty shortages are a national emergency hiding behind professional humility. Here's what faculty would tell you if the system let them be honest:

### 1. Faculty pay is not competitive.

A nurse with a master's degree can make more at the bedside. A nurse with a doctorate can make significantly more in hospital administration.

In other words, we are asking people to take a pay cut to fix the workforce crisis. This misalignment is not incidental—it is baked into how nursing education is funded and valued.

### 2. Faculty workload is overwhelming.

Faculty are teaching, advising, grading, supervising clinicals, managing simulation labs, handling accreditation, conducting program evaluation, rewriting curriculum, mentoring students, serving on committees, and helping with NCLEX prep.

The workload is enormous and unrecognized in most policy discussions.

### 3. Faculty are aging.

Many faculty are nearing retirement, and there is no coordinated national effort to replace them. This is not a pathway problem but a capacity design flaw.

## THE CLINICAL PLACEMENT BOTTLENECK

You cannot graduate a nurse without clinical hours.

But clinical hours are controlled by hospitals, health systems, long-term care facilities, home health agencies, public health departments, and community clinics.

Each of these settings operates under real staffing, resource, and safety constraints. Supporting students requires capacity for supervision, patient safety, and quality care—all of which are increasingly strained.

Why?

- Units are short-staffed.

- Preceptors are stretched thin.

- Patient acuity is rising.

- Hospitals fear liability.

- Students require oversight that staff don't have time to provide.

The results are

- Colleges compete for limited clinical slots.

- Students travel long distances.

- Programs reduce cohort sizes.

- Partnerships become strained.

This tension is frequently expressed across nursing education and practice settings:

> *"We need more RNs, but we can't take more students." "We need a solution that doesn't rely on the goodwill of already overworked nurses."*

This is the definition of structural misalignment. Education demand and clinical capacity are governed by entirely different incentive systems—and they are no longer in sync.

## SIMULATION: THE INNOVATION THAT STILL ISN'T FULLY FUNDED

Simulation should be part of the solution. But without intentional policy and funding alignment, its potential remains unrealized. For many colleges, simulation labs are outdated, underfunded, inconsistently staffed, not aligned with modern curriculum, and poorly integrated into clinical evaluation.

As one simulation leader described the capacity potential when resources are in place:

> *"With adequate funding, I can teach cohorts of students in ways that would require far more clinical hours in hospital settings."*

Simulation can

- Expand capacity

- Standardize learning

- Reduce reliance on scarce clinical sites

- Support adult learners with flexible schedules

- Prepare students for high-acuity scenarios

- Enhance rural education

But simulation programs require equipment, maintenance, trained educators, time, curriculum integration, policy support, and evaluation systems.

Without investment, simulation remains a Band-Aid instead of an accelerator.


## THE REALITY COLLEGES WANT POLICYMAKERS TO UNDERSTAND

Colleges are remarkably consistent in what they ask policymakers to understand:

*If we want more nurses, funding must match expectations.*

Colleges cannot admit more students without more faculty, more clinical placements, more simulation resources, more partnerships, more space, and more support for students.

You can't grow the workforce on goodwill alone.

Traditional policy approaches often say:

- "Expand seats."

- "Increase class sizes."

- "Fast-track programs."

- But colleges are saying: "We cannot expand into nothing. The infrastructure must come first."

This is why The NEXUS Nursing Framework treats capacity as infrastructure—just like roads, broadband, or public transportation.

## A STORY: THE RETURNING ADULT LEARNER CAUGHT IN THE CAPACITY CRUNCH

During my statewide work, I met a single mother who was doing everything right. She worked full-time, cared for two children, and still maintained excellent grades in all her nursing prerequisites.

She was accepted into a nursing program—a moment she had worked years for. But 2 weeks before the semester began, the school lost access to a clinical site, and her cohort had to be reduced.

She was moved to the following year. Her voice cracked when she said to me:

> *"I can't afford to wait a year. I did everything I was supposed to do—this wasn't about me."*

And she was right. When capacity is fragile, students with the least flexibility bear the greatest consequences.

This is not an isolated story. It is common, it is predictable, and it is preventable—if we treat nursing education as a workforce priority instead of an isolated academic silo.

## REGULATION AND CAPACITY

### Understanding BONs vs. Accreditation: Who Regulates What

Nursing education is governed by two distinct bodies—*state Boards of Nursing (BONs)* and *accrediting agencies*—and understanding their roles is essential for solving the nursing workforce crisis. These two systems operate separately, but both shape capacity, quality, and flexibility.

### State Boards of Nursing (BONs)

- Establish licensure requirements
- Determine clinical hour minimums and simulation limits
- Approve new nursing programs and expansions
- Enforce state-level regulations and discipline
- Ensure programs meet statutory and regulatory standards

BONs focus on *public protection,* ensuring that every graduate—regardless of program type—meets safety and competency standards.

### *Accrediting Agencies (e.g., ACEN, CCNE, NLN CNEA)*

- Evaluate academic quality and outcomes

- Review curriculum, faculty qualifications, and student support

- Approve distance learning modalities

- Assess continuous improvement processes

- Allow programs to maintain eligibility for federal financial aid

Accreditors focus on *academic rigor and continuous quality improvement*, not licensure regulations.

## THE CRITICAL DIFFERENCE

Many key decisions—such as simulation limits, clinical hour requirements, or approval of new campuses—are addressed through state Boards of Nursing rather than accrediting bodies. Conversely, issues such as curriculum redesign, online learning, and faculty ratios are typically governed through accreditation standards, often in coordination with state Board of Nursing requirements. Confusion between the two leads to delayed approvals, unnecessary barriers, and misaligned advocacy.

Solving the capacity crisis requires coordinated reform across both bodies—not one or the other. Fragmented advocacy aimed at only one system will continue to stall progress.

### *Where The NEXUS Nursing Framework Fits In*

The NEXUS Nursing Framework creates the language to explain what colleges and clinical partners already know:

**N—Nursing Education Infrastructure:** If students arrive underprepared, faculty spend more time on remediation, increasing workload and decreasing capacity.

**E—Education Capacity:** Faculty shortages + clinical constraints = limited growth

**X—Cross-sector Mobility:** Adult learners face additional barriers when seats are limited and schedules are rigid.

**U—Universal Digital Access:** Simulation and virtual tools need coordinated investment.

**S—Structural Equity:** Capacity shortages disproportionately affect rural and underserved communities.

When these five elements are misaligned, the system slows down. When they are aligned, the system accelerates.

## POLICY RECOMMENDATIONS

Colleges and clinical partners consistently advocate for

1. **Faculty salary parity programs**—State-funded salary supplements to make teaching competitive with bedside nursing

2. **Dedicated clinical capacity expansion funding**—Provides budgets for hospitals and community partners to train preceptors, take more students, update documentation systems, and expand units used for training

3. **Simulation innovation grants**—To modernize and expand simulation capacity statewide

4. **Regional education–clinical compacts**—Ensure that colleges and hospitals collaborate instead of competing

5. **Workforce-aligned accreditation flexibility**—Not lowering standards but aligning them with workforce needs and modern technology

6. **Adult learner–friendly scheduling**—Evening, weekend, hybrid, and accelerated models

7. **Statewide coordination (instead of everyone working alone)**—To avoid duplication, competition, and inequities

## CLOSING REFLECTION

When I look at the nursing workforce crisis, I see something deeper than the headlines.

I see faculty who stayed late to help a struggling student. I see simulation directors fighting to stretch every dollar. I see CNOs trying to balance patient safety with student placement. I see deans carrying decades of underfunding on their shoulders. I see students—especially adult learners—caught in the middle of a broken bridge.

And I see a system filled with brilliant, committed people being asked to do the impossible with infrastructure that has not kept pace.

This chapter is my way of telling their story, giving policymakers the language to finally understand it.

The workforce crisis isn't about interest. It isn't about endurance. It isn't about calling.

It's about capacity. And until we build it, nothing else will move.

# PART II

# THE SYSTEMS THAT SHAPE US

# CHAPTER 8

# Adult Learners and Working Students

*The Missing Middle of the Nursing Pathway*

P art I established that nursing workforce development requires coordinated infrastructure. Part II examines the three major federal systems—Perkins V, WIOA, and Title VIII—and reveals why their disconnection undermines the pathways we need to build.

If you stand inside any nursing program long enough, you'll realize something important: the average nursing student is not 18 years old.

They are often

- Of different ages

- Parents

- Caregivers

- Career changers

- Community leaders

- People working full-time while going to school

- Professionals who were the first in their family to attend college

- Individuals who delayed their education because life got in the way

These are not the students most workforce policies are designed around. But they are the ones carrying the weight of the nursing profession.

Adult learners make up a huge percentage of the nursing pathway—and yet they are often insufficiently accounted for in federal policy design, state funding formulas, and educational systems.

This is why I call them the "missing middle." They are critical to the workforce—yet structurally invisible.

And when adult learners are overlooked, the entire nursing workforce suffers.

## GLOBAL CONTEXT: ADULT LEARNERS AS A UNIVERSAL WORKFORCE CHALLENGE

What we're experiencing in the United States mirrors a global pattern. The Organisation for Economic Co-operation and Development (OECD, 2023) reports that across member nations, adult learners—particularly those balancing work, caregiving, and education—face systemic barriers in accessing health professions training. The International Labour Organization (ILO, 2020) emphasizes that nontraditional pathways and recognition of prior learning are essential for building resilient health workforces, yet they remain underdeveloped in most countries. The World Bank (2023) notes that workforce development systems worldwide struggle to accommodate learners who cannot follow traditional full-time, daytime educational models. These international challenges validate what U.S. nursing educators have long observed: adult learners are essential to the health workforce, yet our systems—from financial aid to clinical scheduling—are rarely designed with their realities in mind.

## A STORY: THE CNA WHO WAS READY TO BECOME AN RN—BUT THE SYSTEM WASN'T READY FOR HER

In my nursing leadership work, I met a certified nursing assistant (CNA) who had worked the night shift for 8 years. She was a natural leader—brilliant, compassionate, patient, and strong. Her colleagues told her she should be a nurse. Her patients assumed she already was.

- She finally decided to go back to school.

- She applied to a local community college nursing program—and she got in. But then reality hit:

- She worked nights and needed day classes.

- The program offered only day clinicals.

- She needed childcare.

- She had no transportation for early-morning rotations.

- She couldn't afford to quit her job.

- Financial aid didn't cover living expenses.

- The program said she had to be "fully available"—which meant not working.

She told me:

*"It wasn't the academics that stopped me. It was the logistics."*

This is a story repeated across adult learners navigating nursing pathways.

The system wasn't designed for them even though they are essential.

## WHY ADULT LEARNERS MATTER TO THE WORKFORCE

Here's what adult learners bring to nursing:

- Maturity

- Life experience

- Resilience

- Emotional intelligence

- Work ethic

- Cultural humility

- Leadership potential

- Career commitment

- Deep motivation

- A sense of calling

They enrich classrooms. They stabilize the workforce. They fill critical roles. They diversify the profession. They stay in the workforce longer.

Adult learners are the heart of nursing. Yet our policies treat them like exceptions.

### The Structural Barriers They Face

This is where The NEXUS Nursing Framework™ helps make sense of the disconnect.

### N—*Nursing Education Infrastructure*

Many learners—particularly those returning to education after time away or coming from underresourced educational settings—enter nursing pathways without robust science preparation, a pattern consistently observed by nursing educators and reflected in prerequisite course progression.

### E—*Educational Capacity*

Rigid program structures hurt them:

- 8 a.m. classes

- Weekday clinicals only

- Full-time attendance requirements

- Limited evening/weekend options

- Lack of bridge programs

- Faculty shortages that restrict cohort sizes

### X—*Cross-sector Mobility*

This is where adult learners struggle most. The Cross-sector Mobility includes:

- Transportation

- Childcare

- Flexible schedules

- Financial support

- Part-time pathways

- Stacking credentials

- Prior learning credits

- Paid apprenticeships

In most states, this element of workforce infrastructure does not exist.

### U–*Universal Digital Access*

Adult learners may lack

- Laptops

- Broadband

- Simulation exposure

- Digital literacy support

These gaps affect performance.

### S–*Structural Equity*

Adult learners are disproportionately:

- Women

- Parents

- Individuals from underresourced communities

- Those living in rural or remote areas

- Students from low-income households

- First-generation college students

Their barriers are heavier and less visible.

## A STORY FROM A RURAL
## COMMUNITY COLLEGE

A rural community college dean described a common challenge:

> *"My adult students can't get to clinicals because the hospital is 45 minutes away and most don't have reliable cars."*

The program attempted carpools, adjusted schedules, and appealed to the hospital for site flexibility. But without transportation infrastructure, these efforts had limited impact. Again, this was not an academic issue—it was an infrastructure constraint.

## A WORKING MOTHER'S STORY

One student told me she left her program not because she couldn't handle the coursework, but because clinical hours conflicted with her childcare schedule.

She said:

> *"I wasn't going to fail. The program just wasn't built for someone like me."*

Imagine losing a future nurse—a strong one—because she couldn't find a babysitter. This is what happens when policy ignores real life.

## POLICY PROBLEMS THAT
## HURT ADULT LEARNERS

Here are some of the most significant policy challenges adult learners face—many of which are not always visible in workforce design discussions:

### 1. The assumption of "full-time enrollment" is unrealistic.

Many adult learners need part-time or hybrid pathways.

### 2. WIOA wasn't designed for multiyear education.

WIOA prioritizes rapid employment, not multiyear clinical education. This hurts CNA-to-LPN and LPN-to-RN pathways.

### 3. Financial aid rules don't match adult learner realities.

FAFSA does not account for childcare, transportation, reduced work hours, or lost income. Adult learners are expected to absorb these costs independently.

### 4. Clinical schedules assume students don't work.

Programs often require early-morning clinical shifts (e.g., 6 a.m.–2 p.m.), which can be incompatible with night-shift or full-time employment.

### 5. Bridge programs are underfunded.

LPN-to-RN programs are limited. CNA-to-LPN pathways are rare. Paramedic-to-RN programs are inconsistent.

### 6. Prior learning credit systems are not standardized.

Adult learners often repeat content they already know.

## POLICY RECOMMENDATIONS

Here's what would change everything:

- Expand evening and weekend nursing programs.
- Fund paid nursing apprenticeships.

- Align WIOA funding to support long-term healthcare pathways.

- Provide transportation and childcare stipends.

- Standardize prior learning credits for healthcare workers.

- Create stackable credential ladders (CNA → LPN → RN → BSN).

- Support hybrid and online didactic education.

- Remove full-time-only barriers for admission.

- Adult learners don't need special treatment—they need realistic design.

## CLOSING REFLECTION

In workforce development discussions I'm part of, a familiar question often emerges:

*"How do we get more young people into nursing?"*

It is an important question, and the answer starts earlier than most people realize.

We absolutely must strengthen K–12 pathways, expand health science exposure, and make sure students see nursing long before graduation.

And there is more to the answer. We cannot build the nursing workforce of the future without investing in the adults who are serving right now.

The CNAs. The medical assistants. The home health aides. The EMTs.

The parents balancing work and caregiving. The career changers. The community health workers.

The people already doing the emotional, physical, and relational work of caregiving—in facilities, in neighborhoods, and in their own homes.

These adults are not backup options.

They are the backbone of the current system and one of the strongest sources of future nurses.

They are ready. They are willing. They are capable.

What they need is not motivation—they need *systems designed with their realities in mind:* flexible scheduling, transportation support, childcare access, bridge programs, apprenticeships, and financial models that reflect adult responsibilities.

Preparing young people and supporting adult learners are not competing priorities. They are two halves of a complete workforce strategy.

If we want a nursing workforce that is large enough, diverse enough, and strong enough to meet the moment, we must build a system that sees *every pathway*—early talent and experienced caregivers alike—and makes room for all of them to rise.

# CHAPTER 9

# WIOA and Nursing Education

## *Why the Systems Don't Align*

f Perkins V shapes the beginning of the nursing pathway, then WIOA (pronounced "whee-oh-uh") shapes the middle.

WIOA is the federal law designed to help people find jobs, change careers, and gain new skills. In theory, it should be one of the most powerful tools for building the nursing workforce.

But here's the problem:

> **WIOA was never designed for careers that take years of education, clinical training, and licensure.**

### WHAT IS WIOA?

The Workforce Innovation and Opportunity Act (WIOA) is the primary federal workforce development program in the United States. Administered through state and local workforce boards, WIOA provides funding for job training, career counseling, and employment services–primarily focused on rapid workforce entry.

WIOA was designed to help people gain skills quickly and enter the workforce in weeks or months, not years. This creates a fundamental mismatch with nursing education, which requires multiyear training pathways.

WIOA was designed for rapid training programs—short, stackable credentials that lead to quick employment.

Nursing is not quick. And it shouldn't be.

This mismatch creates major challenges for nursing students, especially adult learners, career changers, and people from under-resourced communities.

### GLOBAL CONTEXT:
### THE UNIVERSAL CHALLENGE OF
### ADULT WORKFORCE PATHWAYS

The struggle to align workforce development programs with healthcare education is not unique to the United States. The International Labour Organization (ILO, 2020) has documented how countries worldwide face similar tensions between short-term employment programs and the multiyear pathways required for professional healthcare roles. Adult learners seeking nursing careers encounter structural barriers in nations across income levels—from fragmented training systems to inadequate recognition of prior learning. What distinguishes successful systems is intentional policy design that accommodates the realities of healthcare training timelines, while supporting adult learners' economic needs. The United States has the policy tools to address this misalignment; WIOA simply requires redesign to match the demands of nursing education.

## WHAT WIOA ACTUALLY IS (WITHOUT THE LEGISLATIVE JARGON)

WIOA is a federal program that provides

- Tuition support
- Job training
- Career counseling
- Supportive services (sometimes)
- Short-term credentials
- Access to American Job Centers
- Connections to employment

It is run through state workforce boards, local workforce boards, employment and training offices, and job centers.

Its purpose is simple: help people get jobs quickly. Nursing requires

- Multi-semester clinicals
- Rigorous coursework

- Prerequisites

- Licensure exams

- Hands-on experience

- Critical thinking development

This creates friction between what WIOA funds and what nursing requires.

## A STORY: WHAT WORKFORCE PROGRAMS LOOK LIKE IN REAL LIFE

Nearly 3 decades ago, long before I knew the language of "career pathways" or "mobility infrastructure," I served as the Nursing Director of a home healthcare agency in New Jersey. Our agency partnered with WorkFirst NJ, a statewide initiative designed to increase economic mobility by connecting families receiving public assistance to training and employment.

Every few weeks, I met with workforce center staff to review newly certified home health aide candidates. Many were single mothers, first-time workers, or adults reentering the workforce after significant life disruptions.

Hiring them was the easy part. Helping them keep the job—that was the work.

I mentored CHHAs, CNAs, LPNs, and RNs who juggled child care, transportation barriers, financial stress, health challenges, and the emotional labor of caregiving. We coached through everything: time management, professional expectations, boundary setting, and building confidence in environments that had not always welcomed them.

Some advanced into nursing school. Others became leaders in

their agencies and communities. Every one of them changed the way I understood workforce systems.

What I saw back then reflects ongoing gaps in what WIOA is structured to deliver today:

- Supportive services matter.

- Coaching matters.

- Partnerships matter.

- Flexibility matters.

- Understanding the lives of adult learners matters.

Most importantly, people do not fail workforce programs; workforce programs fail when they are not designed to support people.

That realization is why the Cross-sector Mobility (X) in The NEXUS Framework is rooted in human reality—not policy theory.

## A SECOND STORY: THE ADULT LEARNER CAUGHT BETWEEN TWO SYSTEMS

Throughout my years in nursing workforce development, I've heard this story repeatedly. An experienced healthcare worker—perhaps a medical assistant or home health aide—decides she wants to become an RN. She goes to her local American Job Center for support.

The workforce counselor reviews what's fundable and says:

> *"We can support short-term training that gets you certified quickly. But nursing programs? Those take 2 to 4 years. WIOA isn't designed for that."*

She leaves discouraged—not because she lacked ability, but because the system meant to help her essentially said: "Your goal takes longer than the system can support. You'll need to choose a shorter pathway."

The counselor was doing exactly what the system trained them to do.

This is not an equity-aligned outcome. That is structural misalignment.

## WHY WIOA DOESN'T FIT NURSING (TODAY)

Here are the core issues:

1. **WIOA prioritizes short-term credentials**—6–12 week programs get approved easily; 2–3 year nursing programs do not.

2. **Annual funding cycles conflict with multi-year pathways**—WIOA resets yearly. Nursing school doesn't.

3. **Case managers lack healthcare pathway expertise**—Thus, they unintentionally steer students elsewhere.

4. **Supportive services are inconsistent**—Many nursing students need childcare, transportation, uniforms, test fees, books, and tutoring, and WIOA covers these unevenly.

5. **Eligible Training Provider Lists (ETPLs) exclude nursing programs**—Often for reasons like program length, cost, filled cohorts, or clinical site limitations.

6. **WIOA was built for speed, not sustained career ladders**—Healthcare—especially nursing—requires both.

This is the structural issue The NEXUS Framework calls Cross-sector Mobility.

## THE ELIGIBILITY BARRIER

Most WIOA-funded programs prioritize credentials that can be completed in 6–12 weeks. Nursing education typically requires

- 12–18 months for LPN programs

- 2 years for RN programs

- 4 years for BSN programs

- Plus prerequisites

This timeline mismatch means nursing programs are often excluded from Eligible Training Provider Lists (ETPLs)—even though nursing offers higher wages and greater career mobility than many short-term programs.

The result: Career counselors steer aspiring nurses toward shorter programs like phlebotomy or medical assisting, not because these are better pathways, but because they fit WIOA's funding structure.

## THE CHALLENGE
## WORKFORCE BOARDS FACE

Workforce staff are committed to student success, but they operate within strict structural parameters:

- Federal regulations governing WIOA funding

- State-specific interpretations and guidelines

- Performance metrics tied to speed of job placement

- Limited funding pools

- Mandated employment outcome requirements

The fundamental challenge: WIOA's performance framework is designed for rapid workforce entry (weeks to months), while nursing education requires sustained support over multiple years (2–4 years). This structural mismatch produces predictable outcomes across workforce systems.

Career counselors working within WIOA's constraints often guide aspiring nurses toward shorter healthcare credentials—not because these pathways aren't valuable, but because WIOA's design prioritizes programs that achieve quick employment outcomes. Short-term credentials like CNA, phlebotomy, EKG tech, or medical assisting are each valuable and essential to healthcare delivery.

But for adults whose goal is becoming an RN, WIOA's design creates a funding barrier. The system was never intended to support multiyear professional education pathways.

This reflects a structural misalignment between WIOA's original intent (rapid workforce reentry) and nursing's educational requirements, not a failure of career counselors or a problem with healthcare support roles.

## WHERE WIOA ACTUALLY WORKS FOR NURSING (WHEN USED STRATEGICALLY)

WIOA can work—if used intentionally:

1. **Support for prerequisites**—A&P, Microbiology, Medical Terminology, English, Math

2. **Funding for CNA, PCT, or CMA training**—Entry points into nursing

3. **Supportive services**—Childcare, transportation, books, supplies, uniforms

4. **Bridge programs**—CNA → LPN → RN ladders

5. **Apprenticeships**—Wage subsidies for nurse apprentices

6. **Co-enrollment models**—WIOA + community college + employer sponsorship

These bright spots depend on design, not luck.

## WHERE THE NEXUS FRAMEWORK FITS IN

WIOA sits inside the X of The NEXUS Nursing Framework—**Cross-sector Mobility**. Mobility is not just movement. It is

- Financial mobility

- Academic mobility

- Schedule mobility

- Geographic mobility

- Career mobility

WIOA can support all of these—when aligned with nursing programs, healthcare employers, workforce boards, K–12 CTE pathways, and community organizations.

When aligned, nursing pathways flourish. When misaligned, students fall through the cracks.

## POLICY RECOMMENDATIONS

To make WIOA work for nursing, states should:

1. Expand WIOA to support multi-year nursing pathways— Nursing education requires sequenced coursework and clinical training that extends beyond short-term timelines.

2. Increase inclusion of nursing programs on Eligible Training Provider Lists (ETPLs)—Inclusion expands access to WIOA-funded supports for nursing students.

3. Stregnthen training for WIOA case managers in healthcare pathways—Informed navigation improves alignment between workforce services and nursing education requirements.

4. Scale supportive services for nursing students— Transportation, childcare, books, and exam fees are critical to persistence.

5. Expand apprenticeships and earn-while-you-learn models—Paid training reduces financial barriers for adult learners entering nursing.

6. Scale WIOA–college articulation agreements—Clear agreements streamline transitions from workforce programs into nursing education.

7. Strengthen alignment between WIOA, Perkins V, and Title VIII—Alignment across federal programs reduces gaps at key transition points.

8. **Expand part-time enrollment**—Flexibility enables working adults to progress through nursing programs without losing support.

## CLOSING REFLECTION

Nursing students juggle work, school, caregiving, clinical schedules, financial stress, and family responsibilities. The question is never whether they are capable but whether our systems are designed for the lives they actually live.

WIOA can be one of the most powerful engines of mobility—if we reshape it to meet the realities of nursing education.

This chapter is not simply about policy. It is about building a workforce system that sees students not as job placements, but as future nurses, leaders, and healers.

# CHAPTER 10

# Title VIII

*The Federal Investment That*
*Keeps Nursing Education Alive*

I f Perkins V shapes the beginning of the pathway and WIOA shapes the middle, then Title VIII is the lifeline that keeps the nursing education system from collapsing.

Title VIII is the primary federal funding source for nursing education in the United States—a funding stream that consistently supports:

- Nursing faculty development
- Scholarships for students
- Advanced practice programs
- Diversity initiatives
- Public health nursing
- Workforce distribution in rural and underserved areas

While federal accountability discussions continue to evolve, no final determination has been made regarding nursing's classification under federal loan regulations. The purpose of this section is not to predict federal action but to contextualize why funding stability matters for the nursing workforce.

## A NOTE ON THE CHANGING
## FEDERAL LOAN LANDSCAPE

As of this book's publication (January 2026), the federal student loan landscape for nursing education is in a period of significant transition. Recent discussions within the federal rulemaking process—including updates to Financial Value Transparency (FVT) rules—have raised concerns among educators and policymakers about how nursing programs may be classified for federal loan purposes. One proposal under debate involves adjusting the definition of "professional degree" programs, which could change how much federal student aid nursing students are eligible to access.

Although no final policy has been enacted, the implications are substantial. Nursing education is inherently costly: simulation technology, clinical placements, faculty ratios, and extended program lengths all contribute to expenses that exceed those of most undergraduate programs. Many nursing students already graduate with considerable debt. If loan availability were reduced—particularly for pre-licensure students—access to nursing education could narrow further, disproportionately affecting lower-income students, first-generation college students, and communities of color.

Any reclassification that lowers federal loan caps would shift enormous pressure onto states, institutions, and employers to fill the gap. States would be expected to expand loan repayment programs, scholarships, and faculty support at the exact moment the workforce shortage is most acute. This is why cross-sector funding coordination is not merely beneficial—it is essential. When one federal funding stream contracts, other pathways must expand, or the pathways into nursing becomes constrained.

Readers should continue to monitor federal actions related to student loan eligibility and program classifications, as the policy landscape may shift significantly over the coming years.

Without Title VIII, schools would struggle to recruit faculty, modernize programs, expand capacity, support underserved students, sustain advanced practice preparation, and meet community health needs.

Yet, it is a policy that almost no one outside academia or policy circles can explain.

This chapter brings Title VIII down to earth—what it is, why it matters, and how it shapes the future of nursing.

## GLOBAL CONTEXT: HOW NATIONS FUND NURSING EDUCATION

The challenge of adequately financing nursing education is not unique to the United States. The Organisation for Economic Co-operation and Development (OECD, 2023) documents wide variation in how countries fund healthcare workforce training—from direct government subsidy of tuition to employer-sponsored models and hybrid public–private partnerships. The World Bank (2023) emphasizes that sustainable health workforce development requires dedicated, long-term funding mechanisms that support both student access and program quality. Countries that have successfully expanded their nursing workforces—including Norway, Australia, and Canada—have done so through intentional public investment in nursing education infrastructure, faculty development, and student financial support. The United States has such a mechanism in Title VIII, but it remains chronically underfunded relative to workforce need.

## A STORY: THE FACULTY MEMBER WHO STAYED BECAUSE OF A TITLE VIII GRANT

Several years ago, I met a faculty member at a state university who was considering returning to the bedside. Her salary as a nursing instructor was significantly lower than what she could earn in a hospital, and the workload was relentless.

She told me:

*"I love teaching, but I can't sustain this financially."*

Just when she was preparing to resign, the school received a Title VIII faculty loan repayment grant. This grant allowed them to reduce her educational debt, provide development funds, support her role stability, and keep a high-quality educator in the classroom.

She stayed. And because she stayed, dozens of students graduated—students who would go on to fill critical workforce gaps.

That single grant didn't just retain a faculty member. It retained the future workforce. This is Title VIII in real life.

## WHAT TITLE VIII ACTUALLY IS

Title VIII refers to *Nursing Workforce Development Programs* under the Public Health Service Act.

### TITLE VIII AT A GLANCE

Title VIII of the Public Health Service Act is the primary federal funding source for nursing education in the United States.

Administered by: Health Resources and Services Administration (HRSA)

Key programs are

- Nursing Workforce Development Programs

- Nurse Faculty Loan Program (NFLP)

- Nursing Student Loans

- Advanced Education Nursing (AEN) grants

- Nurse Anesthetist Traineeships

- Scholarships for Disadvantaged Students

Without Title VIII, most nursing schools would struggle to recruit faculty, expand enrollment, or support underserved students. It is the backbone of nursing education capacity in the United States.

Administered by the Health Resources and Services Administration (HRSA), Title VIII funds:

- Nursing schools

- Faculty development

- Scholarships

- Loan repayment

- Advanced practice programs

- Entry and advancement pathways that broaden work-force participation

- Nurse-led clinics

- Rural and underserved community placement

Think of it as the federal backbone supporting nursing education.

If Title VIII disappeared tomorrow, nursing schools nationwide would feel it immediately.


## WHY TITLE VIII MATTERS SO MUCH

Here's what Title VIII makes possible:

### 1. Scholarships for students

Especially those from rural communities, minority populations, first-generation backgrounds, and economically disadvantaged backgrounds.

These scholarships are often the difference between staying in school or stopping out.

### 2. Loan repayment for nurse faculty

This part is critical. Faculty shortages are one of the biggest barriers to expanding the nursing workforce.

Title VIII helps schools recruit, retain , and develop faculty, and compete with hospital salaries.

### 3. Support for Advanced Practice Registered Nurses (APRNs)

Nurse practitioners, nurse midwives, clinical nurse specialists, nurse anesthetists—all crucial for expanding access to care.

Title VIII expands access to primary care, maternal health services, rural healthcare, and chronic disease management by funding APRN education and supporting workforce distribution to underserved areas. HRSA placement data documents Title VIII graduates serving in shortage areas, and National Academy of Medicine research validates that APRN practice improves health outcomes, although fragmented data systems make it difficult to measure Title VIII's isolated impact.

### 4. Distribution of the workforce

Title VIII programs place nurses in underserved communities, shortage areas, community health centers, and public health departments.

### 5. Innovation in nursing education

Schools use Title VIII funds to modernize curriculum, add simulation, strengthen clinical partnerships, redesign pathways, and expand enrollment.

Title VIII is the federal lever that allows nursing education to grow.

## WHY TITLE VIII IS OFTEN UNDERRECOGNIZED IN WORKFORCE POLICY

In state and national workforce policy discussions, a common question emerges:

*"Nursing gets such a small share of federal workforce funding. Why is that?"*

Several structural factors help explain this:

- Title VIII is small compared to the size of the problem.

- It competes with numerous other federal priorities.

- Nursing education doesn't have the same visibility as medical education.

- Many policymakers don't understand nursing career pathways.

- The return on investment isn't immediate—it takes years.

But here's why that mindset is dangerous:

*We cannot produce more nurses without investing in the people who teach nurses.*

This is the workforce lever that changes everything.

## WHERE THE NEXUS NURSING FRAMEWORK FITS IN

Title VIII lives at the intersection of E (**Educational Capacity**) and S (**Structural Equity element**) in The NEXUS Nursing Framework.

### E—*Educational Capacity*

Title VIII directly increases capacity by supporting faculty, expanding programs, modernizing equipment, and funding clinical sites. HRSA program data documents these outputs, and nursing education research shows correlation between faculty support and enrollment capacity. While program-level data exists, system-level tracking of Title VIII's aggregate capacity impact remains limited due to fragmented reporting.

### S—*Structural Equity*

Title VIII improves equity by funding underserved students, placing APRNs in shortage areas, reducing financial barriers, and strengthening public health.

**Without Title VIII, both capacity and equity collapse.**

## A STORY FROM A RURAL COLLEGE

In a conversation with a dean of a rural community college, she shared:

> *"Title VIII kept our program alive during a faculty shortage. We were down to two instructors for 90 students."*

Through Title VIII-funded faculty loan repayment, they recruited new faculty, stabilized their team, prevented program shutdown, maintained accreditation, and continued producing nurses for a medically underserved region.

This is what Title VIII does—consistently and essentially.

## POLICY RECOMMENDATIONS

To strengthen Title VIII's impact

1. **Expand funding for faculty loan repayment**—Faculty shortages are the biggest choke point.

2. **Increase scholarships for underserved students—**Especially those from Black, brown, rural, and low-income communities.

3. **Strengthen support for APRN programs—**To expand primary care, maternal care, and rural access

4. **Modernize Title VIII for the digital era—**Allow funding for simulation innovation, virtual learning, and AI-integrated curriculum.

5. **Embed cross-sector alignment—**Encourage coordination among Title VIII, Perkins V, WIOA, HRSA, state workforce boards, and hospitals and health systems.

6. **Make Title VIII part of broader workforce planning—**It is not a standalone line item but a workforce lever.

## CLOSING REFLECTION

Title VIII may not make headlines. It may not be widely understood. It may not feel as urgent as burnout or staffing crises.

However, it is foundational.

Title VIII is the quiet, steady investment that allows faculty to teach, students to persist, programs to expand, rural communities to receive care, and advanced practice nurses to serve where they are needed most.

The nursing workforce does not grow because people are interested in nursing. It grows because the systems that support nursing education are funded, stable, and aligned.

Title VIII is one of those systems.

This chapter is about honoring that truth—and building the workforce we know is possible.

# CHAPTER 11

# HRSA and
# Federal Levers

## *How Federal Agencies Shape*
## *the Nursing Ecosystem*

f you ask many nurses about the Health Resources and Services
Administration (HRSA), you may hear a range of responses:

- "I've heard of it ... I think?"

- "Don't they do something with underserved
  communities?"

- "Aren't they the ones who run nurse loan repayment?"

- "Is that the clinic in my town with the sliding fee scale?"
  Each of these reflects a piece of HRSA's role—but not
  the full picture.

HRSA is one of the most important federal engines supporting
health access, nursing education, community clinics, and workforce
development nationwide.

Yet HRSA often works behind the scenes—quietly ensuring that underserved communities have health centers, nursing students receive scholarships and loan repayment, rural communities have providers, maternal and child health programs exist, public health departments get resources, advanced practice nurses can serve in shortage areas, and primary care is accessible.

If Title VIII is the nursing education lifeline, HRSA is the backbone of equity in healthcare delivery.

This chapter breaks down what HRSA does, why it matters, and how it fits The NEXUS Nursing Frameworkthrough the lens of real stories and workforce realities.

## GLOBAL CONTEXT: HRSA'S MODEL AND INTERNATIONAL INFLUENCE

While HRSA is a uniquely American institution, its model of targeted health workforce investment has influenced international technical assistance programs worldwide. The World Health Organization (WHO, 2020) has worked with countries across income levels to develop analogous systems that link workforce training to underserved community placement—drawing on lessons from programs such as the Nurse Corps and the National Health Service Corps. The Organisation for Economic Co-operation and Development (OECD, 2023) notes that effective health workforce policy requires dedicated agencies that can coordinate across education, employment, and service delivery sectors—precisely what HRSA was designed to do. What makes HRSA's approach particularly valuable is its integration of financial incentives (loan repayment, scholarships) with infrastructure support (community health centers, rural health programs) to ensure that training translates into equitable workforce distribution. This model offers replicable insights for nations working to address their own healthcare workforce shortages and geographic maldistribution.

## A STORY: THE COMMUNITY CLINIC THAT SURVIVED BECAUSE OF HRSA

Early in my career, I worked at a Federally Qualified Health Center (FQHC)—the kind of place where one waiting room, a handful of exam rooms, and a small team carried the weight of an entire community. Later, I also worked in women's health, serving patients who relied on low-cost, accessible care in ways that shaped how I understood equity and public health.

At the FQHC, a nurse practitioner underscored a reality we all recognized:

> *"Without HRSA, this clinic wouldn't exist. And without this clinic, many of our patients would have nowhere else to go."*

That wasn't an exaggeration. For countless people, the FQHC was the only place where they could receive sliding-scale care, chronic disease management, reproductive health services, public health education, and behavioral health support.

And nurses weren't just caregivers. They were translators and advocates—stability in a system with very few safety nets.

I still remember a colleague saying:

> *"We don't just take care of patients. We hold the entire community steady."*

That is the quiet, consistent impact of HRSA-funded care. It's not flashy. It doesn't make headlines. But it stabilizes communities every single day.

## WHAT HRSA ACTUALLY DOES

HRSA invests in

- Workforce training

- Nursing education

- Primary care access

- Maternal & child health

- Community health centers (FQHCs)

- Rural health programs

- Loan repayment & scholarships

- HIV/AIDS programs

- Public health infrastructure

- Provider distribution

Think of HRSA as the federal agency that ensures healthcare reaches people who need it most. It functions through grants, programs, and national initiatives that often feel invisible—but without which the entire workforce system would collapse.

## WHAT IS HRSA?

The Health Resources and Services Administration (HRSA) is a federal agency within the U.S. Department of Health and Human Services.

HRSA's mission: Improve health outcomes and achieve health equity through access

to quality services, a skilled health workforce, and innovative, high-value programs.

HRSA administers:

- Community Health Centers (FQHCs)

- National Health Service Corps

- Title VIII Nursing Programs

- Nurse Corps Scholarship and Loan Repayment

- Ryan White HIV/AIDS Program

- Maternal and Child Health programs

- Rural health initiatives

- Health workforce data and analysis

HRSA funding reaches approximately one in five Americans annually through its network of grantees and programs.

## HOW HRSA SHAPES
## THE NURSING WORKFORCE

HRSA supports the nursing workforce through a range of targeted investments, including:

1. **Title VIII nursing workforce programs** (covered in the previous chapter)

2. **Nurse Corps Loan Repayment Program**, which helps nursing faculty, nurses working in shortage areas, and advanced practice nurses reduce educational debt

3. **Scholarship programs for nursing students**, particularly those from low-income or resource-limited communities

4. **Training grants for nurse practitioners and midwives**, including support for primary care, behavioral health integration, community-based clinical training, and maternal health initiatives

5. **Grants to expand behavioral health nursing**, addressing a rapidly growing workforce need

6. **Public health nursing programs** that strengthen disease prevention, chronic care, health education, and community outreach

7. **Rural health initiatives** that support nurses practicing in geographically isolated communities

8. **Faculty development initiatives** that help colleges recruit, prepare, and retain nursing educators

Taken together, HRSA's investments create a connective infrastructure that links nursing education to community health needs.

## A STORY: THE NURSE PRACTITIONER
## WHO RETURNED HOME BECAUSE OF HRSA

A nurse practitioner shared her story at a statewide workforce roundtable:

She grew up in a rural town. No hospital. Few healthcare resources. No local primary care.

She left to train as a nurse, eventually becoming an APRN. She wanted to return to her hometown to serve—but the debt was overwhelming.

HRSA's Nurse Corps Loan Repayment Program changed everything. She said:

> *"The loan repayment was the only reason I could come back home. HRSA didn't just support my career. They helped me serve my community."*

Today, she is the only full-time primary care provider in that region. Her work reduces ER visits, increases preventive screening, and connects families to needed resources.

That is the ripple effect of HRSA investment.

### Where Is HRSA in The NEXUS Nursing Framework

HRSA sits inside **S—Structural Equity**, but it touches all five elements.

**N—Nursing Education Infrastructure:** HRSA funds training exposure in community health settings.

**E—Educational Capacity:** HRSA supports faculty development and APRN training programs.

**X—Cross-sector Mobility:** Loan repayment, scholarships, and career ladders help adult learners advance

**U—Universal Digital Infrastructure:** HRSA funds telehealth expansion, critical for rural nursing education and care delivery.

**S—Structural Equity:** This is HRSA's core mission: underserved communities, rural access, maternal health, community health centers, and behavioral health.

HRSA is the federal equity engine that makes nursing distribution possible.

## WHY HIGHER EDUCATION DEPENDS ON HRSA MORE THAN MOST REALIZE

Colleges rely on HRSA programs to

- Build APRN programs
- Establish community-based clinical sites
- Hire faculty
- Expand simulation
- Support underrepresented students
- Place trainees in underserved communities
- Meet accreditation standards

Without HRSA, nursing schools shrink, clinical sites disappear, faculty shortages worsen, and access gaps widen.

We cannot talk about nursing capacity without talking about HRSA.

### Federal Levers Beyond HRSA

HRSA is the largest federal player in nursing workforce development, but several other agencies shape the pathway:

**Department of Education**—financial aid, Pell Grants, student success funding, TRIO programs, accreditation oversight

**Department of Labor**—apprenticeships, WIOA, workforce boards, job center systems

**Centers for Medicare and Medicaid Services (CMS)**—reimbursement policies, telehealth coverage, value-based care incentives, quality measures

Together, these agencies influence staffing models, training requirements, reimbursement for nursing services, innovation funding, and pathway alignment.

The future nursing workforce depends on greater interagency alignment rather than siloed policymaking.

This is exactly what The NEXUS Nursing Framework calls for.

## POLICY RECOMMENDATIONS

To strengthen HRSA's impact

1. **Increase funding for Nurse Corps loan repayment and scholarships**—Particularly for faculty and providers in shortage areas.

2. **Expand Title VIII to support nursing faculty salaries—** Faculty capacity remains a primary constraint on program growth.

3. **Increase funding for rural clinical training sites—**APRNs, BSN students, and public health nurses need community-placement models.

4. **Strengthen HRSA–Department of Education partnerships—**Align nursing program investments with financial aid modernization efforts.

5. **Strengthen HRSA–Department of Labor alignment—** This is done so that apprenticeships and WIOA-funded services better align with nursing pathways.

6. **Scale HRSA-supported telehealth training initiatives—** Digital readiness is essential.

7. **Increase HRSA support for behavioral health nursing—** Given the national crisis, this is urgent.

### CLOSING REFLECTION

Like all essential infrastructure, HRSA's work is most visible in its absence. It doesn't trend on social media or capture headlines—but every nursing school, rural health clinic, and community health center in America bears its influence. HRSA is the quiet force behind

- The nurse who returns home to serve

- The community clinic that keeps its doors open

- The nursing faculty member who stays in education

- The student who finishes their degree

- The patient who receives care in an underserved region

This chapter is about honoring that force—and shining a light on the federal levers that make nursing possible. If nursing is infrastructure, then HRSA is one of the pillars that holds it up.

# CHAPTER 12

# State Innovation

*What Policy Leadership Actually Looks Like*

When people talk about "the nursing shortage," they often talk as if the entire country is experiencing the same problem in the same way. But anyone who has worked across states—in policy, education, or nursing leadership—knows the truth:

> *The U.S. nursing infrastructure crisis is national, but the specific gaps vary by state.*

Each state struggles with a different combination of

- Workforce needs
- Healthcare landscape
- Rural/urban realities
- Education policies
- Funding structures
- Regulatory barriers

- Political pressures

- Economic drivers

And because of that, each state innovates differently.

## GLOBAL CONTEXT: DECENTRALIZATION AS A UNIVERSAL CHALLENGE

What we're experiencing in the United States mirrors challenges documented worldwide by the Organisation for Economic Co-operation and Development (OECD, 2023). The OECD's analysis of health workforce policies across member countries reveals that decentralized governance—where regions or states control education, licensing, and workforce planning independently—creates both innovation opportunities and coordination challenges. Countries from Germany to Australia face similar tensions between national workforce needs and local policy control. The World Health Organization (WHO, 2020) notes that this fragmentation often contributes to the global nursing shortage projected to reach 6 million by 2030, as workforce planning becomes reactive rather than strategic.

Here's what makes the U.S. unique: our 50-state system creates 50 natural laboratories for innovation. While fragmentation poses challenges, it also generates policy experiments that can inform national strategy.

Some states are ahead of the curve. Some are holding steady. Some are stuck.

And some are quietly building models the rest of the country should be studying.

This chapter explores state-level innovations that are reshaping the nursing pathway—and what they reveal about the future.

## A STORY: HOW ONE SMALL STATE CLOSED CLINICAL GAPS BY THINKING BIG

In one northeastern state, a community college consortium faced severe clinical shortages. Hospitals were at capacity. Faculty were stretched thin, and student waitlists grew longer each semester.

Instead of competing, the colleges took a strategic approach: they partnered.

Together, they created a statewide clinical coordination center—a centralized, system-level structure that:

- Tracks clinical site availability
- Assigns placements equitably
- Reduces duplication
- Eases hospital scheduling
- Supports simulation alternatives
- Identifies gaps across regions

A nursing dean reflected:

> *"Before, we spent hundreds of hours calling hospitals individually. Now the system works for us—not against us."*

The results were measurable:

- Waitlists dropped
- Faculty workloads stabilized
- Students accessed more consistent clinical experiences
- Hospitals felt less burdened
- Programs were able to expand

This is what happens when states address workforce challenges at the **systems level**—by investing in coordination, shared infrastructure, and collective solutions rather than isolated fixes.

## STATE INNOVATION AREAS THAT REFLECT SYSTEM-LEVEL DESIGN PRINCIPLES

The following innovation areas illustrate how states operationalize alignment across education, workforce, and healthcare systems. While the specific strategies vary, each reflects shared design principles that strengthen nursing workforce capacity over time. These examples are illustrative rather than exhaustive.

### Innovation Area 1: Faculty Recruitment and Retention

Faculty shortages remain one of the most significant constraints on nursing workforce expansion. States that address this bottleneck directly create immediate and durable capacity.

### EXAMPLES:

#### North Carolina—Faculty Loan Repayment Program

- Provides up to $20,000 per year for nursing faculty

- Targets community college and university educators

- Prioritizes underserved and rural areas

#### Texas—Faculty Salary Supplements

- Offers competitive salary support

- Helps programs recruit and retain educators

- Reduces the pay gap between faculty and clinical practice

**Minnesota—Clinical Education Redesign**

- Funds faculty development

- Supports innovation in clinical education

- Helps redesign curricula to reflect modern practice models

**LESSON:**

States that invest directly in nursing faculty expand education capacity and strengthen workforce sustainability.

### Innovation Area 2: Simulation-Based Capacity Expansion

Simulation has emerged as one of the most effective state-level strategies for addressing clinical placement constraints when paired with quality standards and faculty support.

**EXAMPLES:**

**Washington State—50% Simulation Option**

Allows up to 50 percent of required clinical hours to be replaced with high-quality simulation under specific conditions, expanding statewide capacity.

**Florida—Statewide Simulation Funding**

Invested in technology, equipment, and faculty training and established regional simulation centers accessible to multiple nursing programs.

**California—Virtual Simulation Grants**

Supports the integration of virtual and augmented reality into nursing education.

**LESSON:**

Simulation expands enrollment capacity when states invest thoughtfully in infrastructure, faculty preparation, and regulatory alignment.

### Innovation Area 3: K–12 Health Pathways and Dual Enrollment

States that invest early in health career exposure and academic alignment strengthen nursing pathways long before students enter higher education. International research from OECD countries demonstrates that integrated education-to-workforce systems support health profession development. While U.S. data systems do not systematically track K–12 exposure to nursing enrollment, state-level initiatives suggest similar patterns domestically.

**EXAMPLES:**

**Tennessee–Statewide Health Science Pathways**

- Fully funded health science pathways

- Dual enrollment partnerships

- Health science teacher training

- Robust HOSA participation

**Colorado–Career Academies**

- State grants for high school career pathways

- Industry partnerships with healthcare systems

- Transportation and student support services

- Stackable certificates

**Maryland–P-TECH Health Pathways**

- Students graduate with both a high school diploma and an associate degree

- Strong employer partnerships

- No-cost dual enrollment

**LESSON:**

When states invest in early exposure and academic alignment, conditions strengthen for robust nursing pathways well before college entry.

## Innovation Area 4: Apprenticeships and Earn-While-You-Learn Models

Apprenticeship models expand access for adult learners by integrating education, employment, and income—reducing financial barriers while supporting persistence.

**EXAMPLES:**

**Wisconsin–CNA-to-LPN Apprenticeship**

- Paid, structured apprenticeship

- WIOA-funded support

- Employer wage subsidies

- Pathway into RN programs

**Colorado and Kentucky–RN Apprenticeships**

Enable students to work and learn simultaneously under structured supervision.

### Arkansas–LPN-to-RN Apprenticeship

- Accelerated pathway
- Hospital partnerships
- Rural student focus

### LESSON:

When students can earn while they learn, adult learners are more likely to enroll, persist, and complete nursing pathways.

### *Innovation Area 5: State Workforce Compacts and Collaboratives*

Cross-sector alignment is uncommon, but when states invest in formal coordination structures, workforce transformation accelerates.

### EXAMPLES:

### Massachusetts–Nursing Workforce Center

- Tracks workforce data
- Coordinates education and employer needs
- Advises policymakers
- Supports statewide simulation standards

### Wyoming–Cross-Sector Workforce Coordination

- State workforce board (WWDC) coordinating WIOA strategy aligned with education and employer needs
- WIOA-supported workforce centers and grants connecting training to in-demand jobs
- Healthcare Workforce Task Force with cross-agency and education/employer participation

- Coordination of high-demand training (including nursing support roles) with workforce services

## Georgia—Healthcare Industry Partnerships

- Regional workforce boards
- Higher education alignment
- Employer-led collaboration

## LESSON:

Workforce change occurs most rapidly when states align education, labor, and healthcare through sustained governance and coordination.

### *Innovation Area 6: Behavioral Health and Public Health Nursing Investments*

Given growing behavioral health and community health needs, some states are intentionally reimagining nursing pathways beyond hospital-centered models.

## EXAMPLES:

### Oregon—Behavioral Health Scholarships

Supports nursing students preparing for psychiatric and mental health roles.

### Arizona—Public Health Nursing Fellowship

Places BSN students in community health settings to build experience in prevention and population-based care.

### Illinois—Community Health Nursing Initiative

- Nurse-led clinics

- Mobile health units

- Community-based nursing pathways

**LESSON:**

States that invest in behavioral health and public health nursing pathways expand access, strengthen equity, and align the nursing workforce with community needs.

## HOW THE NEXUS NURSING FRAMEWORK™ HELPS STATES INNOVATE SYSTEMICALLY

The most effective states use a NEXUS-aligned approach across all five elements:

**N—Nursing Education Infrastructure:** Early pathways, dual enrollment, K–12 investment

**E—Educational Capacity:** Faculty salaries, simulation funding, clinical alignment

**X—Cross-sector Mobility:** Apprenticeships, stackable credentials, adult learner support

**U—Universal Digital Access:** VR, telehealth, statewide digital tools, broadband access

**S—Structural Equity:** Rural investment, scholarships, diversity initiatives, public health programs. When states align all five elements, transformation becomes possible.

## INTERNATIONAL EXAMPLES

While U.S. states innovate independently, other countries offer models of coordinated state/federal approaches:

- **Australia:** State-federal nursing workforce compacts
- **Germany:** Länder coordination on nursing education
- **Canada:** Provincial health workforce planning councils

These models demonstrate that regional innovation and national coordination aren't mutually exclusive (OECD, 2023).

## POLICY RECOMMENDATIONS FOR STATES

States should

1. **Create statewide nursing workforce councils:** Cross-sector collaboration prevents duplication and inequity.

2. **Invest in faculty through loan repayment & salary incentives:** Faculty shortages are the #1 bottleneck.

3. **Expand simulation and VR capacity statewide:** This should be especially done in rural and under-resourced regions.

4. **Strengthen K–12 health pathways:** Dual enrollment, labs, career academies, and aligned curricula.

5. **Prioritize apprenticeships and earn-while-you-learn models:** Remove financial barriers for adult learners.

6. **Modernize regulation to support innovation:** Allow simulation, hybrid learning, and competency-based models.

7. **Build strong public health and behavioral health pathways:**
   Align with community needs and workforce gaps.

## CLOSING REFLECTION

States don't have to wait for federal reform. They don't have to wait for national consensus. They don't have to wait for perfect alignment. They can act now—and many already are.

State policy innovation shows us something profound: when states invest in nursing as infrastructure, communities thrive. When they don't, communities struggle.

The future of nursing will not be shaped by one federal law or one national initiative. It will be shaped by the states that decide to lead.

# PART III

# MAKING IT REAL

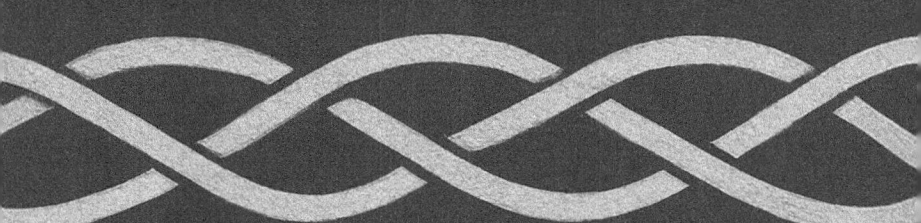

# CHAPTER 13

# Cross-Sector Collaboration

## *The Missing Ingredient*

We've identified the infrastructure gaps and examined the disconnected federal systems. Part III presents a roadmap—how to align these systems, who must lead, and what coordinated action looks like in practice.

If you've ever sat in a meeting with educators, workforce leaders, nursing faculty, hospital executives, and policymakers all in the same room, you already know one thing:

> *Everyone cares deeply. Everyone is trying. And almost no one is speaking the same language. This is the hidden barrier in the nursing workforce crisis:*

We don't have a shortage of passion, willingness, or programs. We have a shortage of alignment.

Nursing is shaped by

- K–12 schools

- Community colleges

- Universities

- Hospitals

- Long-term care facilities

- Public health departments

- Workforce boards

- State agencies

- Federal agencies

- Community organizations

- Philanthropy

- Local government

- Industry partners

However, these systems are organized around different rules, incentives, priorities, and timelines. Everyone owns a piece of the solution, but no one owns the whole thing.

## GLOBAL CONTEXT: THE UNIVERSAL CHALLENGE OF SILOED SYSTEMS

This fragmentation isn't uniquely American. The Organisation for Economic Co-operation and Development (OECD, 2023) documents what they call "ministry silos" across health workforce systems worldwide, where education, health, labor, and finance ministries each control different pieces of the nursing pathway without coordinated oversight. The International Labour Organization (ILO, 2020) reports that these institutional silos are among the most significant barriers to effective nursing workforce development globally. Even in countries with national healthcare systems, coordination between education providers, healthcare employers, and workforce planners remains persistently weak.

What makes this challenge particularly acute in the U.S. is the number of players involved: we have federal, state, and local agencies all operating with different mandates, plus private sector employers, independent educational institutions, and philanthropic organizations. The complexity is exponentially greater but so is the innovation potential.

This chapter pulls back the curtain on what cross-sector collaboration really looks like and how we can design it better.

## A STORY: FIVE LEADERS, ONE PROBLEM, ZERO ALIGNMENT (AT FIRST)

Through my work at the Institute for Health & Social Equity (IHSE), I spent several years in conversation with leaders across education, healthcare, and workforce systems to better understand why the nursing shortage felt so immovable. During that period, I had a series of professional conversations with leaders from across the nursing workforce ecosystem, including:

- A community college dean

- A hospital Chief Nursing Officer

- A K–12 CTE director

- A workforce board leader

- A public health nurse leader

They all named the same problem: "We don't have enough nurses." Everyone agreed on the symptom.

But when I asked what it would take to change it, the misalignment became clear.

A K–12 education leader focused on health career preparation told me: "We can't expand our high school health pathways without updated labs and equipment."

The community college dean said:

> *"We can't take more students without more faculty. We're at capacity."*

The hospital chief nursing officer explained:

> *"We can't handle more clinical students right now. Our staff are overwhelmed."*

A workforce board leader added: "

> *WIOA limits us to funding short-term training. We can't support longer nursing programs."*

And the public health nurse leader added:

> *"Everyone is focused on hospitals. Meanwhile, our communities need more public health and community-based nurses."*

Every leader was right. None were wrong. But none could move the system forward on their own. What I heard was five accurate truths—with zero structural alignment behind them.

This is what the nursing workforce ecosystem looks like before integration: everyone working hard, everyone seeing a different slice of the problem, and no shared framework to bring the pieces together.

## THE FIVE LANGUAGES
## OF NURSING WORKFORCE

Every sector speaks a different language:

- **K–12** speaks in terms of *pathways, exposure, readiness, career preparation, Perkins, and students.* The focus is on early preparation and orientation to the field.

- **Higher education** speaks the language of *capacity, accreditation, faculty, clinical sites, and simulation.* The focus is on quality, standards, and constraints.

- **Hospitals** speak in terms of *staffing, turnover, onboarding, and patient safety.* The focus is on immediate workforce needs.

- **Workforce boards** speak the language of *employment outcomes, WIOA, and performance metrics.* The focus is on job placement and funding rules.

- **Public health** speaks in terms of *community needs, prevention, access, and equity.* The focus is on population-level health.

Everyone is touching the same elephant—but from different angles. The NEXUS Nursing Framework provides a shared language, allowing these sectors to see the whole system rather than isolated parts.

## WHAT TRUE CROSS-SECTOR
## COLLABORATION LOOKS LIKE

When it's done well, collaboration looks like this:

### 1. Shared Problem Definition

Everyone agrees on the same diagnosis, which is not "We need more nurses" but "We need an aligned system that supports K–12 exposure, higher ed capacity, adult learner mobility, digital readiness, and equitable access."

### 2. Shared Data

Partners use

- Common dashboards
- Shared workforce projections
- Regional needs analysis
- Student outcomes
- Clinical capacity mapping

### 3. Shared Incentives

These are not:

- Hospitals funding their own programs
- Colleges competing for clinical sites
- K–12 working in isolation

These are the shared goals, such as

- Regional workforce stability
- Equitable access
- Sustainable capacity
- Local economic development

### 4. Shared Governance

These include statewide or regional councils with

- Educators
- Employers
- Policymakers
- Workforce boards
- Community leaders
- K–12

### 5. Shared Resources

Such as

- Simulation centers
- Clinical placement systems
- Dual enrollment agreements
- Apprenticeship structures
- Faculty development grants

When systems stop competing and start coordinating, everything moves faster.

## A STORY: HOW ONE REGION TURNED COMPETITION INTO COLLECTIVE IMPACT

In a southern state, three community colleges competed for the same clinical sites. Hospitals were overwhelmed by the duplication, and programs were frustrated by unpredictable placements.

So, the region created a Clinical Placement Collaborative. Together they

- Shared clinical schedules
- Distributed placements evenly
- Standardized expectations
- Created joint simulation experiences
- Collaborated on faculty development
- Aligned precepting models

A CNO told me:

*"For the first time, we feel like partners—not gatekeepers."*

This is what cross-sector collaboration can create: relief instead of pressure, partnership instead of competition.

## WHERE CROSS-SECTOR COLLABORATION BREAKS DOWN (PATTERNS I SEE ACROSS STATES)

Through my work in public health, nursing leadership, equity initiatives, and cross-sector interviews, one pattern keeps surfacing: every sector is working hard, but very few are working together.

Not because leaders don't care—they do.

It is because the architecture of our education and workforce systems was never designed for shared ownership.

Across conversations with K–12 educators, college leaders, employers, and workforce partners, the same challenges appear again and again:

### 1. Everyone is fixing their own piece—no one is fixing the connections.

Each sector focuses on its part of the pathway; the linkages between them remain unaddressed.

### 2. Funding streams operate in silos.

Perkins funds K–12. WIOA funds adult learners.

Title VIII funds nursing schools. CMS drives employer behavior. HRSA funds clinics and APRNs.

These programs were never designed to work in concert—and they don't.

### 3. No single entity owns the full education-to-workforce pathway.

Not K–12.

Not higher education.

Not employers.

Not workforce boards.

Each holds one segment, but no one is accountable for the whole.

### 4. Incentives conflict across systems.

Hospitals need staff immediately.

Colleges require high-quality clinical placements.

Workforce boards are measured on rapid job placement.

K–12 systems focus on long-term career exploration.

Public health prioritizes community-centered investment.

These priorities are governed by different timelines and accountability structures, and they frequently operate at cross-purposes.

**5. *Leadership turnover erases institutional memory.***

Leaders transition. Partnerships fade. Momentum stalls.

What begins as collaboration often becomes fragmentation.

This is what The NEXUS Nursing Framework identifies as structural misalignment—not a failure of commitment, but a failure of connection.

### INTERNATIONAL EXAMPLES

Some countries have addressed cross-sector fragmentation through:

- **Netherlands:** National nursing workforce councils with education, employer, and government representation

- **Singapore:** Ministry of Health coordinates healthcare workforce planning with education ministry

- **Ireland:** Single national body oversees health workforce development from K–12 through continuing education

These models show that coordination requires dedicated infrastructure, not just goodwill (OECD, 2023).

### Design Principles and What They Enable in Practice

States that make measurable progress on nursing workforce challenges do not rely on isolated programs. Instead, they apply a consistent set of design principles, which show up in different ways depending on local context.

### 1. Dedicated, Operational Governance

**Principle:** Effective states establish governance structures focused exclusively on nursing pathways that are empowered to coordinate across sectors.

**What this enables in practice:**

- Statewide nursing workforce centers or collaboratives
- Formal mechanisms to align education, employers, workforce boards, and public health
- Sustained leadership beyond grant cycles

*Illustrated by:* Massachusetts Nursing Workforce Center; Georgia Healthcare Industry Partnerships.

### 2. Shared Data as System Infrastructure

**Principle:** Strong systems treat data as shared infrastructure, not as proprietary or siloed information.

**What this enables in practice:**

- Workforce forecasting tied to education capacity
- Better alignment between faculty supply, clinical placement, and employer demand
- Policy decisions informed by real-time system constraints

*Illustrated by:* Massachusetts workforce tracking; simulation standards linked to capacity planning; performance metrics used by workforce boards.

### 3. Backbone Infrastructure for Coordination

**Principle:** States invest in backbone organizations that provide continuity, coordination, and accountability across institutions.

**What this enables in practice:**

- Regional collaboratives that support multiple schools and employers

- Faculty development and simulation standards shared across programs

- Stable leadership that holds long-term strategy, not just individual initiatives

*Illustrated by:* Nursing workforce centers; regional simulation hubs; multi-institution collaboratives.

### 4. Coordination as a Funded Function

**Principle:** Successful states fund coordination itself—not just programs—recognizing that systems do not run automatically.

**What this enables in practice:**

- Faculty recruitment and retention programs that align education and funding policy

- Shared simulation centers accessible to multiple schools

- Apprenticeships that coordinate employers, educators, and workforce funding

*Illustrated by:* Faculty loan repayment and salary support (NC, TX); statewide simulation investments (FL, WA, CA); earn-while-you-learn apprenticeship models.

### 5. Policy Alignment as a Core Design Element

**Principle:** Rather than treating policies as separate levers, effective states intentionally align education, workforce, and healthcare policy so incentives point in the same direction.

**What this enables in practice:**

- Faculty investments that complement, rather than conflict with, workforce funding

- Apprenticeships supported by both education and labor policy

- Regulatory flexibility (e.g., simulation allowances) paired with quality standards

*Illustrated by:* Alignment across Perkins-supported pathways, WIOA-funded apprenticeships, state regulation, and employer incentives—without requiring a single linear sequence.

### 6. Equity by Design, Not by Exception

**Principle:** High-performing systems design for rural and underserved communities from the outset rather than retrofitting equity later.

**What this enables in practice:**

- Faculty incentives targeting underserved regions

- Transportation, support services, and earn-while-you-learn models for adult learners

- Pathways into behavioral health and public health nursing aligned with community needs

*Illustrated by:* Rural-focused apprenticeships (AR); transportation supports (CO); behavioral and public health nursing investments (OR, AZ, IL).

### How The NEXUS Nursing Framework™ Supports Collaboration

The five elements of NEXUS provide a common architecture for cross-sector work:

**N—Nursing Education Infrastructure:** K–12 leaders see their role in early preparation

**E—Educational Capacity:** Higher ed and clinical partners coordinate training capacity

**X—Cross-sector Mobility:** Workforce boards and employers support adult pathways

**U—Universal Digital Access:** Technology partners expand access

**S—Structural Equity:** All partners prioritize equity and rural access

When every partner understands how their work connects to all five elements, silos begin to dissolve.

## POLICY RECOMMENDATIONS

To make cross-sector collaboration real, states and regions must:

### 1. Create regional nursing workforce councils

With clear authority and operational responsibility—not advisory roles.

### 2. Fund coordination

Invest in dedicated staff to manage partnerships, convene stakeholders, and align systems.

### 3. Build shared data systems

- Clinical capacity maps
- Pathway and progression dashboards
- Learner mobility tracking
- Equity and access indicators

### 4. Align funding streams across agencies

Braid education, labor, health, and higher education investments to support continuity.

### 5. Require employer partnerships in funding proposals

Hospitals, long-term care, and public health partners should be embedded in program design.

### 6. Develop statewide clinical coordination platforms

Reduce competition, streamline placement, and expand clinical capacity.

### 7. Design regionally responsive models for rural and resource-limited communities

- Mobile and shared simulation resources
- Regional education and clinical hubs
- Telehealth-enabled training and digital infrastructure

## CLOSING REFLECTION

Cross-sector collaboration is not a meeting, a task force, or a press release. It is the ongoing, committed, often difficult work of aligning systems that were never designed to work together.

But when it happens—when educators, employers, policymakers, and communities truly align—everything changes:

- Capacity expands

- Access improves

- Burnout decreases

- Retention strengthens

- Students persist

- Communities thrive

The nursing workforce is not rebuilt by any single system. It is rebuilt by systems working as one.

# CHAPTER 14

# The New Workforce Ecosystem

*Designing for the Future We Want*

I f you've made it this far in the book, you already know something
fundamental: The nursing workforce we have is the result of the
systems we built. The nursing workforce we need is the result of the
systems we design.

Right now, our systems are producing

- Shortages

- Burnout

- Misalignment

- Inequity

- Bottlenecks

- Confusion

- Preventable barriers

But none of this is inevitable. It is the result of design.

The future of nursing is not about hoping things get better. It is about building an ecosystem where nurses, students, educators, communities, and employers can all thrive.

## GLOBAL CONTEXT: WORKFORCE ECOSYSTEMS AS STRATEGIC PRIORITY

The concept of workforce ecosystems, rather than simple pathways, aligns with international best practices. The World Bank's Human Capital Project (2023) emphasizes that effective health workforce development requires coordinated systems connecting education, employment, and community support structures. The World Economic Forum's Future of Jobs Report (2023) identifies healthcare as a sector where ecosystem thinking is essential: no single institution can produce the workforce needed, but coordinated networks can. Various countries, from South Korea to Germany, have moved beyond linear training models to create what the OECD (2023) calls "learning ecosystems"—dynamic networks that support workers throughout their careers.

What the U.S. brings to this global conversation is scale and complexity. Our challenge is greater, but our capacity for innovation across diverse settings is unmatched.

This chapter is about that future—what it looks like, why it matters, and how we design it.

## A STORY: THE DAY A HEALTH SYSTEM REALIZED "WE CAN'T FIX THIS ALONE"

During a strategic workforce summit, I watched a hospital leader present a slide that showed

- Rising nurse vacancy rates

- Shrinking applicant pools

- Decreased retention

- Longer onboarding times

- Increased travel nurse reliance

He paused, looked around the room filled with educators, K–12 leaders, public health officials, and workforce boards, and said:

> *"We cannot hire our way out of this problem. We have to build our way out."*

In that moment, the conversation shifted from individual organizational strategies to a shared acknowledgment that solving workforce challenges would require coordinated action across systems—including:

- K–12

- Community colleges

- Universities

- Public health

- Workforce boards

- Government

- Community organizations

And perhaps most importantly, he added:

> *"We need a system that doesn't collapse every time someone leaves."*

That moment captured the challenge ahead: moving from isolated efforts toward a more resilient workforce ecosystem built through coordination across systems.

## WHAT IS A WORKFORCE ECOSYSTEM?

A workforce ecosystem is a connected system of education, training, support, policy, technology, and community structures that make it possible for people to enter, stay in, and advance in a profession.

For nursing, this includes

- K–12 pathways

- Community colleges

- Universities

- Hospitals

- Public health

- Long-term care

- Workforce boards

- Community clinics

- Philanthropy

- Policy makers

- Digital infrastructure

- Equity support

When these systems are connected, students flow smoothly. When they are disconnected, students struggle.

The nursing workforce ecosystem must be designed with alignment, equity, and modernization in mind.

## THE FUTURE WORKFORCE ECOSYSTEM HAS 10 ESSENTIAL FEATURES.

These are the qualities this book is leading readers toward—the blueprint for the world we want to build:

### 1. Seamless K–12 → College → Career Pathways

No broken links. No unknowns. No unnecessary barriers.
Just clear, supported, intentional movement.

### 2. Faculty as an Essential Workforce

Competitive salaries. Loan repayment. Professional development. Long-term investment.

### 3. Clinical Capacity Modernized Through Simulation & Partnerships

Simulation isn't supplemental—it is infrastructure. Clinical sites are coordinated and equitably distributed.

### 4. Apprenticeships & Learn-While-You-Earn Models

Adult learners no longer choose between feeding their children and becoming nurses.

### 5. Digital & AI-Ready Curriculum

Students understand

- Telehealth

- Data literacy

- Virtual care

- AI clinical support tools

This is essential for modern practice.

### 6. Universal Workforce Data Systems
Shared dashboards for

- Student movement

- Clinical capacity

- Workforce supply/demand

- Equity indicators

- Retention

### 7. Equity Built Into Every Stage
It is not an add-on, not an afterthought, but a foundational design principle.

### 8. Public Health + Behavioral Health Integrated
Nurses are trained for prevention, community care, and whole-person health.

### 9. Cross-Sector Governance
It includes permanent, resourced, statewide or regional bodies that coordinate the ecosystem.

### 10. Sustainable Funding Models
Perkins, Title VIII, WIOA, HRSA, state funding, philanthropy—aligned, braided, and targeted strategically.

This is the ecosystem The NEXUS Nursing Framework anticipates.

## INTERNATIONAL EXAMPLES

Several countries offer models of integrated workforce ecosystems:

- **Denmark:** "Flexicurity" model connects education, employment support, and retraining throughout careers.

- **Singapore:** SkillsFuture initiative creates lifelong learning pathways with employer co-investment.

- **Switzerland:** Dual education system integrates work and learning from secondary education through professional development.

These models suggest that coordinate approaches strengthen workforce outcomes compared to fragmented systems (OECD, 2023 World Bank, 2023).

## WHERE THE NEXUS NURSING FRAMEWORK™ FITS INTO THE FUTURE ECOSYSTEM

The NEXUS Nursing Framework becomes the architecture of the ecosystem:

**N—Nursing Education Infrastructure:** We build robust K–12 and college systems that prepare students for modern nursing.

**E—Educational Capacity:** We invest in faculty, simulation, clinical partnerships, and high-quality programs.

X—**Cross-sector Mobility:** Students, especially adult learners, can enter and advance without unnecessary barriers.

U—**Universal Digital Access:** Digital tools connect systems and improve learning and care.

S—**Structural Equity:** No community is left behind.

Rural. Urban. Underserved. Underfunded.
This alignment transforms fragmentation into coherence.

### What It Takes to Build This Ecosystem

This is where systems thinking, leadership, and policy converge. States and regions must

1. **Design nursing as a workforce ecosystem, not a pipeline.** Pipelines are linear. Ecosystems are dynamic.

2. **Fund backbone organizations.** Coordination cannot be volunteer-driven.

3. **Build modern simulation & VR infrastructure.** This is capacity, not luxury.

4. **Create true dual enrollment health pathways.** Students should finish high school with momentum, not confusion.

5. **Align WIOA, Perkins, and Title VIII.** Braided funding creates stability.

6. **Expand apprenticeships for adult learners.** This is an equity strategy.

7. **Integrate public health & behavioral health.** The future workforce must be community-ready.

8. **Partner with philanthropy.** Foundations often fund innovation before government does.

9. **Build rural and underserved health systems into planning.** Equity requires design, not hope.

10. **Hold healthcare employers accountable as co-creators.** They should not be only consumers of talent but also co-investors in talent.

This is how we rebuild the workforce for the next generation.

### How the Five Elements Support Ecosystem Design

Each element of NEXUS strengthens the ecosystem

- **Nursing Education Infrastructure (N):** Creates early awareness and preparation.

- **Educational Capacity (E):** Ensures quality training at scale.

- **Cross-sector Mobility (X):** Enables career advancement and adult entry.

- **Universal Digital Access (U):** Leverages technology for reach and quality.

- **Structural Equity (S):** Embeds fairness from design through delivery.

When all five elements function together, the ecosystem becomes self-sustaining rather than crisis driven.

## CLOSING REFLECTION

The nursing workforce crisis is not a failure of individuals—it is a failure of systems. And systems are not fixed by blame; they are fixed by design.

The future workforce ecosystem is within reach. We have the tools, the partners, the data, and the frameworks. We have examples of what works—and the urgency to act.

# CHAPTER 15

# Families, Communities, & Faith Institutions as Workforce Builders

Policymakers often describe nursing pathways through a systems lens—focusing on education structures, funding mechanisms, and regulatory frameworks that shape workforce development.

Nurses, when reflecting on their own journeys, often tell a different story—one centered on the people and communities who helped them persist.

Both perspectives matter. Systems create opportunity, but relationships sustain it.

Nurses describe support that looks like this:

*"My mom watched my kids."*

*"My church helped me pay for books."*

*"My community believed in me."*

*"My grandmother prayed me through."*

*"My youth group leader handed me a scholarship application."*

*"My neighbor drove me to clinicals."*

*"My pastor encouraged me not to give up."*

This reflects an often-overlooked reality of the nursing workforce: families, faith institutions, communities, mentors, and informal support systems are frequently the difference between a student persisting through a pathway or stepping away.

Policies matter. Funding matters. Pathways matter.

But without community scaffolding, even the strongest formal systems often struggle to support students through the hardest parts of the journey.

## GLOBAL CONTEXT: COMMUNITY AS SOCIAL INFRASTRUCTURE

The recognition of community support as essential workforce infrastructure aligns with international research. The World Bank's Human Capital Project (2023) emphasizes that formal education systems succeed or fail based on the strength of surrounding social infrastructure—families, community organizations, and cultural institutions that provide mentorship, encouragement, and practical support. The International Labour Organization (ILO, 2020) documents how community-based support systems are particularly crucial for adult learners and first-generation professionals navigating career transitions. Research across OECD countries shows that students from strong community networks have significantly higher completion rates in health professions, regardless of socioeconomic background (OECD, 2023).

What's distinctive about the U.S. context is the diversity and strength of community institutions—from faith communities to neighborhood organizations to family networks—that can be mobilized for workforce development when formally engaged as partners.

This chapter explores community-level infrastructure—the ecosystem that surrounds the student long before they enter a classroom and long after they graduate.

## A STORY: THE GRANDMOTHER WHO BECAME PART OF THE WORKFORCE PATHWAY WITHOUT KNOWING IT

During a listening session, a young nurse shared how she completed her RN program as a single mother. She said:

> *"I didn't drop out because my grandmother stepped in. She watched my baby on clinical days. She drove me when my car broke down. She sat with me while I studied. She told me that being a nurse was my calling. She kept me going."*

Her grandmother didn't know anything about:

- NCLEX prep
- Faculty shortages
- Clinical placements
- State policy
- Title VIII
- Accreditation

But she kept the pathway alive.

This is what community infrastructure looks like.

### *Community as Workforce Infrastructure*

We rarely talk about community in workforce planning, but the truth is that the nursing workforce is built in living rooms, churches, corner stores, barber shops, community centers, and kitchens—long before it is built in classrooms.

Communities are where students learn

- Identity

- Confidence

- Discipline

- Values

- Resilience

- Work ethic

- Service

- Calling

- Persistence

Communities are where students find

- Encouragement

- Accountability

- Mentorship

- Networking

- Belonging

- Hope

These are not soft supports. They are foundational workforce supports.

You cannot separate community from career.

Not in nursing. Not in any human-centered profession.

## FAITH COMMUNITIES: AN OVERLOOKED SOURCE OF LEADERSHIP AND SUPPORT

In my own life, faith has always shaped my sense of purpose and direction. Long before I stepped into nursing, public health, or policy work, it was my faith community that nurtured my confidence, affirmed my calling, and reminded me that I was created for impact.

What I've learned, both personally and through the students and leaders I've mentored, is this: faith communities often play a quiet but powerful role in

- Encouraging purpose and identity

- Affirming calling and direction

- Offering scholarships and financial support

- Supporting mental, emotional, and spiritual well-being

- Cultivating early leadership skills

- Providing mentorship and guidance

- Creating intergenerational support networks

And yet, they are almost never invited into workforce development conversations. That absence is a missed opportunity.

Faith-based organizations have the capacity to strengthen student success and career pathways in very practical ways. They can

- Host weekend or summer health science experiences
- Sponsor scholarships or emergency funds
- Partner with nursing or public health programs
- Offer mental health and wellness support
- Match students with mentors
- Assist with transportation or childcare
- Create encouragement circles and small groups
- Host community health events
- Organize tutoring or study groups
- Provide quiet, safe spaces for studying

For many young people—especially those navigating environments where opportunities are limited—faith communities are often the first place they are truly seen, supported, and encouraged to imagine a bigger future.

### INTERNATIONAL EXAMPLES

Here are some international examples of community-driven workforce support:

- **Brazil:** Faith-based health worker training programs in underserved favelas

- **Kenya:** Community health worker programs supported by local churches and mosques

- **India:** Women's self-help groups providing mutual support for nursing students

These models demonstrate that formal workforce systems achieve better outcomes when they partner with existing community institutions rather than replacing them (WHO, 2020; World Bank, 2023).

## FAMILIES: THE ORIGINAL WORKFORCE DEVELOPERS

Families—in all forms—are the earliest shapers of career identity. They

- Encourage (or discourage) career aspirations
- Model work values
- Provide emotional stability
- Support study time
- Offer transportation
- Help with childcare
- Celebrate milestones
- Advocate for students

A student may enter nursing because

- An auntie was a caregiver
- A cousin urged them to pursue healthcare
- A parent saw their gift for compassion
- A sibling encouraged their dreams

Family support isn't just emotional—it's structural. Families are workforce infrastructure.

## COMMUNITY ORGANIZATIONS:
## THE MISSING MIDDLE

Community groups—nonprofits, mentorship programs, student clubs, YMCAs, afterschool programs—often act as connectors between

- K–12
- Colleges
- Employers
- Families

Through my work at the Institute for Health & Social Equity (IHSE)

- Scholarships
- Mentorship
- Leadership development
- Purpose formation

These small interventions create long-term impact. Community organizations can

- Help students complete prerequisites
- Build study cohorts
- Provide financial support
- Connect students to clinical exposure
- Offer career coaching
- Guide students through application processes

- Support adult learners
- Host workshops and info nights
- Build local health talent pathways

They are the glue that holds the ecosystem together.

## HOW THE NEXUS NURSING FRAMEWORK™ INCORPORATES COMMUNITY

Each element of NEXUS depends on community strength:

**N—Nursing Education Infrastructure:** Community organizations introduce K–12 students to healthcare careers through exposure events, mentorship, and early encouragement.

**E—Educational Capacity:** Families and faith communities provide the childcare, transportation, and emotional support that enables students to complete training programs.

**X—Cross-sector Mobility:** Community networks help adult learners navigate career transitions, offering practical support during vulnerable transition periods.

**U—Universal Digital Access:** Community spaces (libraries, faith centers, community centers) provide internet access and study space for students without reliable home resources.

**S—Structural Equity:** Community organizations specifically serve populations that formal systems often miss—offering culturally responsive support, language assistance, and advocacy.

Community infrastructure doesn't replace formal systems—it makes formal systems actually work for real people.

## WHAT POLICYMAKERS AND EDUCATORS CAN DO

To strengthen community-level workforce infrastructure,

### 1. Formally recognize community partners in workforce planning

Include family support services, faith organizations, and community groups in regional workforce councils.

Fund community-based support services such as transportation, childcare, emergency funds, and mentorship programs—these aren't extras; they're necessities.

### 2. Create partnership models between colleges and community organizations

Formalize relationships so community groups can guide students through application processes, provide coaching, and offer wraparound support.

### 3. Support family engagement programs

Help families understand nursing pathways, financial aid, and how to support student success.

### 4. Engage faith communities strategically

Create partnerships with churches, synagogues, mosques, temples, and other spiritual communities that serve student populations.

### 5. Build scholarship and emergency fund infrastructure

Community organizations need resources to provide timely financial support when students face unexpected barriers.

### 6. Create mentorship networks

Connect nursing students with community members who have successfully navigated similar pathways.

### 7. Design for cultural relevance

Recognize that communities support their members in different ways and ensure policy frameworks allow for locally responsive solutions.

## CLOSING REFLECTION

The nursing workforce is not built only in classrooms and hospitals. It is built in living rooms and church basements. In barbershops and corner stores. In grandmother's kitchens and youth group meetings. In conversations over coffee and prayers before exams.

Community infrastructure is often less visible at the policy level—but deeply felt by students who rely on it to persist. If we want to build a nursing workforce that reflects and serves our communities, we must invest in the communities themselves. Not as afterthoughts, not as "nice-to-haves," but as essential partners in workforce transformation.

The NEXUS Nursing Framework recognizes this truth: the five elements of nursing workforce infrastructure cannot function without the sixth—community. And when properly supported and engaged, community becomes the foundation on which everything else is built.

# CHAPTER 16

# Leadership for the Next Generation

*The Attributes, Mindsets, and Skills Tomorrow's Nurses Will Need*

When we talk about the nursing workforce of the future, we often focus on numbers:

- How many nurses do we need?

- How many faculty?

- How many seats in programs?

But numbers alone don't build a workforce. *People do. And people need leadership.*

And it is not leadership defined by titles, seniority, or positional power. Leadership for the next generation of nurses will look different—because healthcare is changing, communities are changing, and the world is changing.

## GLOBAL CONTEXT: THE UNIVERSAL NEED FOR NURSING LEADERSHIP

The challenge of developing nurse leaders is not unique to the United States. The World Health Organization (WHO, 2020) has identified leadership development as a critical component of health workforce strengthening globally, noting that countries with robust nursing leadership frameworks demonstrate better health outcomes and stronger pandemic preparedness. The International Council of Nurses (ICN, 2021) emphasizes that leadership capacity at all levels—from bedside to boardroom—is essential for addressing global health priorities including universal health coverage, health equity, and workforce sustainability. This international consensus validates that the leadership attributes outlined in this chapter reflect universal needs within nursing, even as implementation strategies must be adapted to local contexts.

Tomorrow's nurses will need a new set of attributes, mindsets, skills, and spiritual grounding to thrive. Through stories, insights, and the lived realities nurses face every day, this chapter outlines exactly what those are.

## A STORY: THE NEW NURSE WHO LED BEFORE SHE REALIZED IT

A newly graduated nurse I met at a conference once told me she didn't think she was a leader.

"*I'm too new,*" she said. "*I don't have a title. I'm still learning.*"

But then she shared that during a chaotic shift, when everyone was overwhelmed, she

- Checked on the anxious family members

- Made sure her colleagues took breaks

- Reassured a student nurse who felt unprepared

- Advocated for a patient who needed pain medication

- Escalated a change in condition that prevented deterioration

She didn't realize those were leadership behaviors because she imagined leaders as directors, presidents, managers, and administrators.

But leadership is not positional. Leadership is relational. Leadership is ethical. Leadership is human. That nurse was already a leader—she had simply not been told she was one.

The next generation must be taught to see leadership this way.

## LEADERSHIP IS NOT POSITIONAL

Traditional views equate leadership with titles and hierarchy. But nursing leadership begins at the bedside:

- **Relational:** Building trust with patients, families, and colleagues

- **Ethical:** Advocating for what is right, even when it's difficult

- **Human:** Seeing people, not just tasks or protocols

*The next generation must be taught to recognize leadership in their everyday actions not just in corner offices.*

### Leadership Attribute #1: Purpose Driven

Tomorrow's nurses must know *why* they are here. Not just "I want a stable career" or "I want to help people" but a deeper understanding of calling, values, identity, mission, and service.

Purpose helps nurses stay grounded in their work, especially amid complex and demanding systems. Purpose is the anchor that keeps nurses grounded.

Tomorrow's workforce needs that same clarity.

### *Leadership Attribute #2: Systems-Oriented Thinkers*

- Nurses of the next generation must be able to see beyond the bedside into the system:

- What policies shape patient care?

- How do education and workforce systems interact?

- How does public health affect clinical practice?

- How do inequities shape outcomes?

They must understand care coordination, social drivers of health, workforce dynamics, technology integration, and community ecosystems.

The nurses who thrive will be those who can connect dots—across sectors and systems.

### *Leadership Attribute #3: Collaborative*

The future of healthcare is team-based. Tomorrow's nurses must

- Collaborate across disciplines

- Communicate across cultures

- Partner with patients

- Serve on cross-sector teams

- Build community alliances

- Work with educators and policymakers

Collaboration is not optional. It is a core competency for the future.

### Leadership Attribute #4: Innovation Minded

Not tech obsessed or trend-chasing but curious, creative, open, adaptable.

Nurses must be willing to

- Challenge outdated policies

- Question broken processes

- Design new solutions

- Use technology wisely

- Advocate for modernized systems

Innovation isn't fancy. It's practical. It's courageous. It's the ability to imagine something better.

Tomorrow's nurses need that imagination.

### Leadership Attribute #5: Emotionally Intelligent

Clinical skill matters—but emotional intelligence is what sustains a caregiver.

The next generation must be taught

- Self-awareness

- Perseverance

- Communication

- Conflict navigation

- Empathy

- Boundary-setting

- Mindfulness

- Cultural humility

The most effective leaders are those who can navigate emotion as well as policy.

### Leadership Attribute #6: Advocates

Whether at the bedside or in boardrooms, nurses must be able to speak up for

- Patients

- Colleagues

- Themselves

- Communities facing structural barriers to health and opportunity

- Policy change

Advocacy is not activism alone. It is evidence-informed, equity-driven, system-focused, and strategically communicated.

Nurses must know how to use their voices. The next generation needs that same courage.

### Leadership Attribute #7: Lifelong Learners

The world is changing rapidly. Healthcare is evolving. Technology is advancing.

Tomorrow's nurses will need

- Ongoing training
- Professional development
- Credentialing pathways
- Digital and AI literacy
- Leadership education

Stagnation is no longer an option. Growth is essential.

## THE SEVEN LEADERSHIP ATTRIBUTES

Tomorrow's nurse leaders must be

- **Purpose Driven**—Anchored in calling and values
- **Systems Oriented**—Able to see beyond the bedside
- **Collaborative**—Team-based and cross-sector focused
- **Innovation Minded**—Curious, creative, and adaptive
- **Emotionally Intelligent**—Self-aware and culturally humble
- **Advocates**—Speaking up for patients, equity, and change
- **Lifelong Learners**—Committed to growth and development

*These attributes are not optional—they are essential for thriving in modern healthcare.*

## WHERE LEADERSHIP FITS INTO THE NEXUS NURSING FRAMEWORK™

Leadership is the thread that ties the entire NEXUS Framework together.

**N—Nursing Education Infrastructure:** Students need early leadership development, starting in K–12.

**E—Educational Capacity:** Faculty must model leadership behaviors and teach them intentionally.

**X—Cross-sector Mobility:** Adult learners often bring leadership experiences that must be recognized and valued.

**U—Universal Digital Access**—Leadership is required to integrate new technologies responsibly.

**S—Structural Equity**—Leaders must challenge inequities and design just systems.

Leadership is not a separate topic. It is the foundation that makes The NEXUS Framework real.

## PRACTICAL TOOLS FOR DEVELOPING NEXT-GENERATION NURSE LEADERS

Here are some actionable strategies schools, employers, and communities can implement:

1. **Leadership modules in K–12 pathways**—Based on empathy, service, teamwork, and purpose

2. **Leadership courses in community colleges & universities**— Not just management but leadership as well

3. **Nurse-led mentorship programs**—Pairing graduates with seniors, high schoolers with nursing students, adult learners with peer mentors

4. **Leadership residencies for new graduates**—Layered into clinical onboarding

5. **Faith-based leadership circles**—Especially for students navigating purpose-driven careers

6. **Equity and ethics workshops**—To prepare nurses to lead in diverse communities

7. **Interprofessional leadership training**—Working with social workers, physicians, public health professionals

Leadership must become part of the curriculum, not an elective.

## LEADERSHIP DEVELOPMENT STRATEGIES

**For education:** K–12 leadership modules, undergraduate leadership courses, equity and ethics workshops

**For employers:** Leadership residencies for new grads, nurse-led mentorship programs, interprofessional training

**For communities:** Faith-based leadership circles, peer mentoring networks–Community-based support groups

*Leadership development must be intentional, early, and sustained across the entire nursing journey.*

## CLOSING REFLECTION

Tomorrow's nursing workforce will be asked to carry more than any generation before them, encountering

- Higher acuity patients

- More complex technology

- Deeper inequities

- Public health crises

- Rapid system changes

However, they will also have more opportunity to

- Innovate

- Lead

- Shape the future

- Influence policy

- Redefine care

- Transform communities

Leadership is not a luxury. It is the difference between surviving the profession and shaping it.

This chapter is a call to action—to invest in the leaders we want tomorrow by cultivating them today.

# CHAPTER 17

# Policy Recommendations

*What Leaders Across
the System Must Do Now*

The nursing workforce crisis—and the broader fragility of the health workforce—is not a shortage of people. It is a shortage of alignment.

## GLOBAL CONTEXT: WORKFORCE POLICY COORDINATION WORLDWIDE

The need for coordinated workforce policy is a global imperative. The Organisation for Economic Co-operation and Development (OECD, 2020) reports that healthcare workforce shortages across member countries stem not from lack of interest in health careers, but from fragmented policies across education, labor, and health systems. The International Labour Organization (ILO, 2022) similarly emphasizes that integrated workforce strategies—connecting education ministries, labor departments, and health agencies—consistently outperform siloed approaches in both workforce production and retention.

These international findings reinforce a core premise of this book: workforce challenges persist not because solutions are unknown, but because systems remain misaligned.

Grounded in decades of workforce research, international policy guidance, and community-based practice, the recommendations that follow reflect widely recognized strategies used across systems rather than approaches unique to any single organization. The NEXUS Nursing Framework identifies the system-level levers where action is most urgently needed. What follows is a concise set of recommendations to guide state leaders, policymakers, educators, health systems, workforce partners, and community organizations toward a coordinated response.

## FOR STATE POLICYMAKERS

The following recommendations reflect widely documented best practices in nursing workforce policy, health systems planning, and cross-sector coordination. They are drawn from federal guidance, state innovation efforts, and international workforce frameworks and are intended to support alignment across education, workforce, and health systems.

- Establish statewide nursing workforce councils with cross-agency representation and authority across K–12 education, higher education, public health, workforce development, and Medicaid.

- Invest in nursing faculty capacity through salary parity

initiatives, recruitment incentives, and loan repayment programs aligned with HRSA priorities.

- Expand access to simulation and virtual training infrastructure, including shared regional simulation centers and clinical education hubs.

- Align and braid federal workforce and education funding streams (e.g., Perkins V, WIOA, Title VIII, HRSA) into coordinated, community-serving workforce strategies.

- Modernize licensure and regulatory infrastructure to support innovative education and training models, including apprenticeships, concurrent enrollment, and expanded use of simulation.

- Prioritize rural and underserved regions in nurse training programs, residencies, and workforce incentive initiatives.

- Ensure sustained investment in public health nursing capacity as part of statewide workforce strategies, recognizing its role in prevention, preparedness, and community health resilience.

*These recommendations are intended to strengthen system coordination rather than prescribe a single governance or funding model.*

## FOR HIGHER EDUCATION LEADERS

The following recommendations are grounded in established research on adult learning, workforce mobility, and nursing education capacity. They reflect approaches already in use across multiple institutions and regions and are presented here to support greater alignment and scalability.

- Expand flexible academic pathways, including evening, weekend, and hybrid formats, to better serve working learners and adult students.

- Standardize prior learning assessment (PLA) practices across institutions to accelerate student mobility and reduce unnecessary repetition.

- Increase simulation capacity through investment in trained faculty, evidence-based debriefing models, and shared simulation resources.

- Strengthen clinical partnerships through regional consortia, enabling institutions to share clinical placements, faculty expertise, and preceptor resources.

- Integrate public health, digital health, and AI readiness into nursing curricula to prepare graduates for evolving care delivery environments.

*These strategies focus on expanding capacity and improving alignment across institutions rather than redefining individual program models.*

## FOR K-12 SYSTEMS

The following recommendations reflect widely cited best practices across K–12 education, workforce development, and health career pathway literature. They draw on established policy guidance, cross-sector research, and community-based approaches implemented in various forms nationwide.

- Support the integration of health science pathways in high schools, aligned with community college prerequisites to ensure continuity across the education-to-workforce continuum.

- Strengthen STEM foundations in grades K–8 through inquiry-based learning and age-appropriate, career-connected instruction.

- Reduce counselor caseloads or designate specialized career advisors with expertise in nursing and health career pathways.

- Expand equitable access to dual enrollment coursework, including anatomy and physiology, medical terminology, and English and math readiness.

- Strengthen school–college–employer partnerships, in coordination with local workforce systems, to support mentorship, tutoring, career exposure, and paid work-based learning opportunities.

- Establish formal transition points between K–12 systems and workforce partners, ensuring students in health science pathways are connected to career navigation, work-based learning, and postsecondary workforce supports as they advance.

*These recommendations highlight system-level levers rather than prescribe a single implementation model.*

## Nursing and STEM-Aligned Pathways

Nursing education is science- and technology-intensive. Students pursuing nursing complete rigorous coursework in biology, chemistry, anatomy and physiology, statistics, and increasingly digital health and informatics—requirements comparable to those of many fields traditionally classified as STEM.

Despite this overlap, nursing and health science pathways are not consistently recognized within STEM funding, accountability, and reporting frameworks at the K–12, postsecondary, or workforce levels. This inconsistency has practical implications. STEM designation often influences access to early exposure programs, laboratory investments, dual enrollment opportunities, data reporting, and dedicated funding streams—particularly at the secondary school level.

Recognizing nursing as part of a broader STEM-aligned health career continuum does not require redefining nursing's professional identity. Rather, it ensures that students interested in nursing are not unintentionally excluded from science-focused resources, pathways, and supports that shape preparation and access long before postsecondary education.

Aligning nursing pathways with STEM-related education and workforce frameworks strengthens early preparation, improves continuity across systems, and supports more intentional investment in the science foundation required for nursing education and practice.

## FOR WORKFORCE DEVELOPMENT BOARDS

The following recommendations reflect established practices for aligning workforce funding, supportive services, and career mobility in high-demand sectors such as nursing.

- Authorize multi-year WIOA support for nursing education and training pathways.

- Expand access to supportive services, including childcare, transportation, and technology, to enable persistence among working learners.

- Develop CNA → LPN → RN → BSN apprenticeship and career ladder models in partnership with local employers.

- Seed mobility infrastructure through wraparound supports and community-based career advisors.

- Prioritize nursing as a high-demand, high–return-on-investment sector within local and regional workforce plans.

## FOR HOSPITALS AND HEALTH SYSTEMS

Health systems play a critical role in stabilizing and sustaining the nursing workforce through shared investment and partnership.

- Co-invest in simulation centers and serve as clinical partners in regional education and training networks.

- Expand paid residencies and transition-to-practice programs to improve early-career retention.

- Collaborate on earn-while-you-learn models and tuition-supported pathways for incumbent workers.

- Participate in regional workforce councils to align training capacity with community needs.

- Strengthen preceptor training and recognize precepting as a form of professional leadership.

## FOR COMMUNITY ORGANIZATIONS AND FAITH-BASED PARTNERS

Community-based organizations provide essential mobility supports that formal systems often cannot.

- Provide micro-scholarships to offset costs such as testing fees, scrubs, childcare, and transportation.

- Offer mentoring, study spaces, and basic needs support for students and working learners.

- Coordinate youth exposure programs through partnerships with nurses, hospitals, and educational institutions.

- Strengthen the mobility infrastructure that surrounds students and adult learners as they navigate complex systems.

## WHAT SUCCESS LOOKS LIKE

When policy aligns across the NEXUS elements, we see

- **More students prepared**—K–12 STEM and health pathways produce college-ready candidates.

- **Fewer students turned away**—Faculty investment and simulation expansion increase capacity.

- **Adults able to advance**—WIOA flexibility and stackable credentials enable mobility

- **Technology expanding access**—Broadband, simulation, and AI prepare modern nurses

- **Equity embedded**—Scholarships, wraparound supports, and community partnerships close gaps

*This is the nursing workforce ecosystem our communities deserve.*

## FOR PHILANTHROPY

- Prioritize rural and underrepresented communities in funding decisions.

- Fund innovation pilots that test new models of nursing education and workforce development.

- Support community-based exposure programs that reach students early.

- Invest in data infrastructure that enables cross-sector collaboration.

## POLICY ALIGNMENT PRINCIPLES

Effective nursing workforce policy requires

- **Cross-sector coordination**—Education, workforce, health, and community systems working together

- **Braided funding**—Perkins V, WIOA, Title VIII, and HRSA aligned toward common goals

- **Equity focus**—Rural, underserved, and underrepresented communities prioritized

- **Evidence-based innovation**—Testing new models while scaling what works

*The NEXUS Framework™ provides the structure for this alignment.*

## CLOSING REFLECTION

These recommendations are not aspirational. They are actionable.

Every sector has a role. Every leader has power. Every policy matters.

The nursing workforce will not rebuild itself through market forces alone. It requires intentional design, coordinated investment, and sustained commitment.

The NEXUS Nursing Framework offers the structure. These recommendations offer the path. Now the work begins.

# CHAPTER 18

# Nursing as Calling, Infrastructure, and Shared Responsibility

There is a moment in every nurse's career—sometimes loud and sometimes quiet—when you realize that what you do is more than a job. More than a skillset. More than a role.

It is a calling.

And once you answer that calling, you begin to see the world differently. You see suffering where others see inconvenience.

You see possibility where others see limitation. You see humanity where others see protocol.

You see systems where others see problems, inequity where others see outcomes, leadership where others see hierarchy, and purpose where others see work.

This book has been about seeing—seeing the full system that shapes who becomes a nurse, where they train, how they advance, where they practice, and ultimately, who receives care.

**Global Context: Nursing as Global Health Security**

Countries that invested in nursing infrastructure before COVID-19 saved lives. The WHO (2021) now recognizes nursing workforce capacity as foundational to pandemic preparedness and health system stability. The OECD (2021) documented what we learned the hard way: nations with strong nursing education infrastructure, flexible training models, and workforce mobility mechanisms demonstrated better outbreak responses and lower excess mortality. This is not a domestic workforce issue—it is global security infrastructure.

## WHAT WE HAVE LEARNED

The nursing workforce crisis is not a mystery. It is not an accident. And it is not unsolvable.

It is the predictable result of systems that were never designed to work together—and often never designed with nurses, students, or communities at the center. Throughout this book, we have examined those systems:

In *Part I,* we reframed the crisis. The nursing workforce is not simply a staffing problem to be solved by human resources departments. It is infrastructure—as essential to community well-being as roads, broadband, and clean water. When nursing infrastructure is strong, communities thrive. When it fractures, the cracks spread everywhere: into schools, clinics, rural towns, maternal health, and family stability.

In *Part II,* we traced the systems that shape nurses across their journey—from K–12 classrooms where career identity begins, through higher education where capacity constraints turn away qualified students, into workforce systems where adult learners struggle to find pathways that fit their lives. We examined the federal policies that fund and regulate nursing education: Perkins V, WIOA, Title VIII, and HRSA. We explored state-level innovations and the profound challenge of cross-sector collaboration. At every stage, the pattern was the same—dedicated people working hard inside systems that do not connect.

In *Part III,* we turned toward the future. We envisioned a workforce ecosystem designed with intention—one where K–12 pathways flow seamlessly into higher education, where adult learners can advance without choosing between their families and their futures, where digital tools expand access rather than deepen divides, and where equity is not an afterthought but a design principle. We honored the role of families, communities, and faith institutions as workforce builders. We named the leadership attributes the next generation of nurses will need. And we offered concrete policy recommendations for every sector.

Through it all, The NEXUS Nursing Framework™ provided our organizing structure:

N—**Nursing Education Infrastructure:** Where the pathway begins

E—**Educational Capacity:** Where bottlenecks form

X—**Cross-sector Mobility:** Where adult learners are lost or lifted

U—**Universal Digital Access:** Where the future is built

S—**Structural Equity:** Where justice is either embedded or ignored

These five elements are not separate silos. They are linked. They are interdependent. Weakness in one creates strain across the entire system. Strength in one reinforces all the others.

That is the nexus—the point of connection where everything comes together.

---

**THE NEXUS FRAMEWORK ELEMENTS**

The five interconnected elements that shape the nursing workforce are

- **N—Nursing Education Infrastructure:** K–12 STEM readiness, health science pathways, dual enrollment, early exposure

- **E—Educational Capacity:** Faculty availability, clinical placements, simulation capacity, accreditation

- **X—Cross-sector Mobility:** Stackable credentials, prior learning credit, apprenticeships, wraparound support

- **U—Universal Digital Access:** Simulation labs, broadband access, telehealth readiness, AI literacy

- **S—Structural Equity Element:** Community resources, rural access, scholarships, culturally responsive training

*Weakness in one element creates strain across the entire system. Strength in one reinforces all the others.*

## THE STAKES

Let me be direct about what is at stake.

Without a strong nursing workforce, hospitals cannot function safely. Rural communities lose access to care. Maternal mortality rates climb. Children with chronic conditions go unmonitored in schools. Mental health crises go unmet. Elders in long-term care facilities receive less attention than they deserve. Public health emergencies overwhelm systems built on the assumption that nurses will always be there.

Nurses will not always be there—not unless we build the infrastructure to sustain them. The cost of inaction is not abstract. It is measured in

- Preventable deaths
- Delayed diagnoses
- Exhausted nurses leaving the profession
- Students turned away from programs
- Communities without providers
- Families without support
- Generations of talent never developed

No single sector can address nursing workforce challenges alone; coordinated responsibility is essential.

## THE OPPORTUNITY

And yet, within this crisis lies profound opportunity.

We know what works. We have seen states that invest in faculty and watch their programs grow. We have seen districts that build health science pathways and send students into nursing with confidence and preparation. We have seen workforce boards that redesign WIOA to support multiyear credentials. We have seen hospitals that partner with colleges instead of competing with them. We have seen community organizations that wrap students in support and watch them persist against all odds.

The solutions exist. What we lack is alignment.

The NEXUS Nursing Framework offers that alignment—a shared language, a common lens, a way for educators, employers, policymakers, and community leaders to finally see the same system and work toward the same goals.

This is not idealism. It is pragmatism. Systems that are designed to connect will outperform systems that operate in silos. Investments that are coordinated will yield greater returns than investments that are scattered. Leaders who understand the full ecosystem will make better decisions than those who see only their piece.

The opportunity before us is not merely to produce more nurses. It is to build a workforce ecosystem that is

**Aligned**—Where K–12, higher education, workforce development, and healthcare work as one system

**Equitable** —Where zip code, income, and race no longer predict who becomes a nurse

**Modern**—Where digital tools, simulation, and AI prepare nurses for the healthcare of tomorrow

**Sustainable**—Where faculty are valued, pathways are funded, and nurses can build careers without burning out

**Human**—Where calling is honored, communities are partners, and every student knows someone believes in them

This is the workforce our communities deserve.

## A CALL TO ACTION

Wherever you sit in this ecosystem, you have a role to play.

*If you are a state policymaker,* you have the power to align funding streams, convene cross-sector councils, invest in faculty, and hold systems accountable for outcomes. The NEXUS Framework gives you a map. Use it.

*If you are a higher education leader,* you have the power to expand pathways, modernize curriculum, standardize prior learning credit, and partner beyond your campus walls. Your capacity constraints are real—but so is your influence.

*If you are a K–12 educator or administrator,* you have the power to introduce students to possibilities they have never imagined. You see talent before anyone else does. That is sacred work.

*If you are a workforce board leader,* you have the power to reshape how WIOA serves nursing pathways, to expand supportive services, and to champion apprenticeships that let adults earn while they learn.

*If you are a hospital or health system executive,* you have the power to co-invest in education, expand clinical capacity, build residency programs, and treat workforce development as a strategic priority rather than someone else's responsibility.

*If you are a public health leader,* you have the power to advocate for school nurses, community health nurses, and maternal health programs that are chronically underfunded and deeply essential.

*If you are a community organization or faith-based partner,* you have the power to provide scholarships, mentorship, transportation, childcare, study space, encouragement, and love. Never underestimate how much that matters.

*If you are a student,* you have the power to persist—even when the system makes it hard. And you have the power to change the system once you're through it.

*If you are a nurse,* you have the power to mentor, to advocate, to lead, and to remind everyone why this work matters. Your voice carries weight. Use it.

No single sector can solve this alone. But together—aligned around a shared framework, committed to equity, focused on the future—we can build something that lasts.

---

### YOUR ROLE IN THE NEXUS

Every stakeholder has power to strengthen the nursing workforce:

- **Policymakers** → Align funding, convene councils, invest in faculty

- **Educators** → Expand pathways, modernize curriculum, standardize credit

- **Workforce Leaders** → Reshape WIOA, expand supports, champion apprenticeships

- **Employers** → Co-invest in education, expand capacity, build residencies

- **Communities** → Provide scholarships, mentorship, wrap-around support

- **Students & Nurses** → Persist, mentor, advocate, lead

*The NEXUS Framework™ provides the structure. Your action brings it to life.*

## A PERSONAL REFLECTION

I began this book by sharing that I wrote it because I have watched people try to fix the nursing shortage through quick solutions, isolated interventions, and reactionary policies.

I have also watched something else.

I have watched K–12 teachers see promise in students long before anyone else believed in them. I have watched adult learners study between shifts, after bedtime stories, and before the sun rose. I have watched nurses carry the weight of broken systems on their bodies and still show up with compassion. I have watched faculty stay late, stretch budgets, and pour themselves into students who needed one more chance. I have watched community members offer rides, scholarships, prayers, and meals to students who had no safety net. I have watched policymakers do their best with incomplete information and advocates fight for change year after year.

I have watched people build what they could not yet see. That is the spirit this work requires.

The NEXUS Nursing Framework is my contribution—a way of organizing the complexity, naming the connections, and offering a path forward. But the framework means nothing without the people who use it.

You are those people.

## THE WORK BEFORE US

The nursing workforce will not rebuild itself. Systems do not align by accident. Equity does not emerge from neglect. The future does not arrive—it is built by

- Educators who refuse to accept that some students don't belong in nursing

- Policymakers who choose alignment over turf
- Employers who invest in talent pathways, not just recruitment campaigns
- Communities who wrap their arms around students and refuse to let go
- Nurses who remember what it felt like to be new—and who reach back to help
- Leaders who see the whole system and have the courage to change it

This book has given you the analysis, the framework, the stories, and the recommendations. Now the work is yours.

### THE FUTURE WE ARE BUILDING

The nursing workforce we build today will

- **Honor calling**—Recognizing nursing as more than a job
- **Strengthen infrastructure**—Building the systems that sustain nurses
- **Advance equity**—Ensuring everyone can access nursing careers
- **Embrace innovation**—Using technology to expand rather than replace
- **Foster leadership**—Cultivating the attributes tomorrow's nurses need

*Let us build with intention. Let us build with alignment. Let us build together.*

## CLOSING THOUGHTS

Nursing is more than a profession. It is an infrastructure that holds communities together, leadership that speaks truth to systems, calling that answers when no one else will.

It is equity that demands everyone receive care. It is connection—the nexus—where education, workforce, health, and humanity meet. The workforce we build today will shape the health of generations to come.

Let us build it with intention. Let us build it with alignment. Let us build it with equity at the center. Let us build it together.

The future is calling, and it is time to answer.

*Dr. Sherri Johnson,*
DNP, MPA, RN, FADLN, FAAN

# Strengthening Career and Technical Education for the 21st Century Act

## *(Perkins V)*

## OVERVIEW

The Carl D. Perkins Career and Technical Education Act (Perkins V), signed into law on July 31, 2018 (Public Law 115-224, H.R. 2353), represents the primary federal investment in career and technical education (CTE) in the United States. This reauthorization modernized workforce preparation by strengthening alignment between secondary and postsecondary education, emphasizing evidence-based practices, and expanding access for special populations.

## PURPOSE AND SCOPE

Perkins V provides approximately $1.3 billion annually in federal funding to states to:

- Develop and improve CTE programs at secondary and postsecondary levels

- Strengthen connections between education and workforce needs

- Support programs of study that prepare students for high-skill, high-wage, or in-demand occupations

- Increase access for special populations, including economically disadvantaged students, students with disabilities, and English learners

## KEY PROVISIONS
## AFFECTING NURSING PATHWAYS

**Programs of Study:** Perkins V requires coordinated sequences of courses from secondary through postsecondary education, aligned with industry needs. For nursing, this enables structured pathways from high school health science programs through postsecondary nursing education.

**Work-Based Learning:** The law emphasizes authentic workplace experiences, including clinical rotations, job shadowing, and apprenticeships—critical components of nursing education that Perkins V can support at the secondary level.

**Postsecondary-Secondary Coordination:** Perkins V strengthens requirements for collaboration between high schools and colleges, enabling dual enrollment, early college programs, and articulation agreements that support seamless nursing pathways.

**Special Populations:** The law requires states to describe how they will provide equitable access to CTE for special populations, addressing the structural equity gaps discussed in Chapter 5.

## GAPS IN NURSING WORKFORCE DEVELOPMENT

Despite Perkins V's strengths, significant gaps limit its effectiveness for nursing workforce development:

1. **Funding Ends at Transition Points:** Perkins V support typically concludes when students complete secondary CTE programs or early postsecondary credentials (CNA, LPN). Students pursuing RN licensure—which requires additional prerequisite courses and extended clinical training—fall into a funding gap between Perkins V and Title VIII.

2. **Limited Adult Learner Focus:** While Perkins V serves adult learners through postsecondary institutions, it primarily emphasizes traditional-age students. Adult learners returning to nursing—a substantial portion of the workforce talent stream—face barriers that Perkins-funded programs are not always designed to address.

3. **Disconnection from Clinical Capacity Systems:** Perkins V does not coordinate with healthcare workforce development systems (HRSA, Title VIII) that manage clinical site partnerships, faculty development, or simulation resources essential to nursing education.

## THE NEXUS FRAMEWORK SOLUTION

The NEXUS Nursing Framework™ calls for intentional braiding of Perkins V with WIOA and Title VIII to create continuous support across the full nursing pathway. When states coordinate these funding streams, students can move seamlessly from K–12 health science programs through prerequisite courses and into clinical nursing education without falling through policy gaps.

For policymakers, this means structuring Perkins V Local Applications to explicitly connect with WIOA-supported bridge programs and Title VIII-funded clinical education, ensuring nursing students receive coordinated support at every stage.

### LEGISLATIVE REFERENCE

Public Law 115-224, Strengthening Career and Technical Education for the 21st Century Act, 115th Congress (2017-2018). Available at: https://www.congress.gov/bill/115th-congress/house-bill/2353

# Acronyms and Definitions

## FEDERAL & WORKFORCE POLICY

**CMS (Centers for Medicare & Medicaid Services)**—Federal agency that regulates reimbursement and influences employer behavior

**ETPL (Eligible Training Provider List)**—State-approved list of programs eligible for WIOA funding

**HRSA (Health Resources & Services Administration)**—Federal agency that funds workforce development, community clinics, rural health, and nursing education (including Title VIII)

**Perkins V**—Federal law that funds Career & Technical Education (CTE) in high schools and community colleges. It s shapes early exposure, labs, pathways, and dual enrollment.

**Title VIII**—The main federal nursing education funding stream (scholarships, loan repayment, faculty development)

WIOA (Workforce Innovation and Opportunity Act)—Federal workforce law that funds job training, supportive services, and rapid employment programs through workforce boards

## EDUCATION & CLINICAL TRAINING

APRNs (Advanced Practice Registered Nurses)—Nurse practitioners, nurse midwives, clinical nurse specialists, nurse anesthetists

Clinical placement—Supervised real-world training required for nursing licensure

CTE (Career & Technical Education)—High school and community college programs that prepare students for careers

Dual enrollment—High school students taking college courses that count toward both a diploma and a degree

Simulation (SIM)—Technology-based training that replaces or supplements clinical hours

## NURSING & WORKFORCE TERMS

ADN (Associate Degree in Nursing)—Two-year degree leading to RN licensure

BSN (Bachelor of Science in Nursing)—Four-year degree for RN licensure

FQHC (Federally Qualified Health Center)—Community-based clinics that provide care regardless of ability to pay

**Stackable credentials**—Certificates or degrees that build on each other (CNA → LPN → RN → BSN).

**Mobility infrastructure**—Support systems that help students enter and advance in nursing (childcare, transportation, flexible scheduling, apprenticeships).

# Summary of The NEXUS Nursing Framework™

The NEXUS Nursing Framework *is* a system-level structure for building a modern, equitable nursing workforce.

## N–NURSING EDUCATION INFRASTRUCTURE

- K–12 STEM readiness
- Health science pathways
- Dual enrollment
- Early exposure
- Foundational literacy + numeracy

## E–EDUCATIONAL CAPACITY

- Faculty availability
- Clinical placements
- Simulation capacity

- Accreditation alignment
- Sustained Investment

## X—CROSS-SECTOR MOBILITY

- Pathways for adult learners
- Stackable credentials
- Prior learning credit
- Apprenticeships
- Transportation + childcare
- WIOA alignment

## U—UNIVERSAL DIGITAL ACCESS

- Simulation labs
- Broadband access
- Telehealth readiness
- AI + digital literacy
- Virtual learning

## S—STRUCTURAL EQUITY

- Community resources
- Rural access
- Scholarships + support
- Workforce distribution
- Culturally responsive training

Together, these five elements form the ecosystem that determines

- Who becomes a nurse

- Where they train

- How they advance

- Where they practice

- Who receives care

# Crosswalk of Federal Levers (Perkins V, WIOA, Title VIII, HRSA)

## WHERE IT FITS

| Lever | What It Funds | In NEXUS | Policy Rationale |
|---|---|---|---|
| Perkins V | K–12 + community college CTE, labs, equipment, dual enrollment | N | Builds early exposure and readiness; reduces K–12 inequities |
| WIOA | Adult learners, job training, supportive services | X | Enables mobility for working adults; often misaligned with nursing |
| Title VIII | Nursing scholarships, faculty development, APRN programs | E + S | Supports faculty, expands capacity, supports underserved communities |
| HRSA | Community clinics, rural health, nurse loan repayment, telehealth | S + U | Distributes workforce equitably; strengthens community-based care that supports population health outcomes |

# Critical Breakdown Points in Nursing Pathways: A Stage-by-Stage Infrastructure Analysis

| Stage | Typical Breakdown | Who Is Most Affected |
|---|---|---|
| **Elementary & Middle School** | Limited STEM exposure<br><br>Inconsistent science instruction<br><br>Lack of inquiry-based learning | Students in rural and under-resourced communities<br><br>Students in racial and ethnic communities historically underrepresented in STEM and health career pathways<br><br>Girls in under-resourced STEM environments |

| Stage | Typical Breakdown | Who Is Most Affected |
|---|---|---|
| **High School** | No health science pathways<br><br>Limited dual enrollment<br><br>High counselor caseloads | Students in rural and frontier districts<br><br>Students in under-resourced urban school systems<br><br>Students who are the first in their families to navigate postsecondary education |
| **College Preparation & Prerequisites** | Underdeveloped science foundations<br><br>High D/F/W (Drop, Fail, Withdrawal) rates in A&P or chemistry<br><br>Cost and financial barriers | Students who are the first in their families to navigate postsecondary education<br><br>Students navigating economic resource constraints<br><br>Adult learners returning after academic gaps |
| **Nursing Program Admission** | Capacity limits<br><br>Faculty shortages<br><br>Limited flexible or part-time options | Community college applicants<br><br>Adult learners<br><br>Students balancing caregiving responsibilities |
| **Clinical Training** | Limited clinical placements<br><br>Preceptor shortages<br><br>Transportation or scheduling barriers | Students in rural communities<br><br>Students navigating economic resource constraints<br><br>Working adult learners |

| Stage | Typical Breakdown | Who Is Most Affected |
|---|---|---|
| **Transition to Practice** | High-acuity practice environments<br><br>Inconsistent residency programs<br><br>Underdeveloped onboarding | New graduates<br><br>Nurses from underrepresented backgrounds in high-stress settings |
| **Career Advancement & Mobility** | Limited bridge programs<br><br>Inflexible schedules<br><br>Tuition barriers | Working adults<br><br>CNAs and LPNs<br><br>Nurses practicing in rural and underserved areas |

**Note:** Breakdowns reflect system-level infrastructure gaps rather than individual deficits.

# Policy Recommendations by Sector

## FOR STATES

- Create statewide nursing workforce councils.

- Fund faculty loan repayment and salary parity initiatives.

- Expand statewide simulation infrastructure.

- Align Perkins, WIOA, Title VIII, and HRSA funding streams.

## FOR HIGHER EDUCATION

- Expand hybrid, evening, and weekend pathways.

- Standardize prior learning credit.

- Increase simulation-to-clinical ratios responsibly, consistent with evidence-based standards.

- Build regional clinical placement compacts.

## FOR K-12 EDUCATIONS SYSTEMS

- Integrate health science pathways aligned with community college prerequisites.

- Strengthen K–8 STEM foundations through inquiry-based, career-connected instruction.

- Designate specialized advisors with expertise in nursing and health career pathways.

- Expand equitable access to dual enrollment coursework aligned with postsecondary readiness.

- Strengthen school–college–employer partnerships to support mentorship, career exposure, and work-based learning.

- Establish formal transition points connecting K–12 students to postsecondary education and workforce supports.

## FOR WORKFORCE BOARDS

- Authorize multiyear WIOA support for nursing pathways.

- Train case managers on nursing career pathways.

- Fund apprenticeships and stackable credentials.

- Increase access to supportive services (childcare, transportation).

## FOR HOSPITALS AND HEALTH SYSTEMS

- Co-invest in simulation centers.

- Build earn-while-you-learn models.

- Expand clinical site partnerships.

- Adopt residency models to retain new graduates.

## FOR COMMUNITY ORGANIZATIONS AND FAITH INSTITUTIONS

- Provide micro-scholarships.

- Offer study space, mentoring, and transportation support.

- Host career exposure events.

- Build community support networks.

# Economic Impact Calculation Methodology

The workforce impact calculations presented throughout this book (e.g., *"1 biology teacher = 6 potential nurses"*) are illustrative examples intended to demonstrate order-of-magnitude effects, not precise econometric forecasts. These calculations use conservative assumptions grounded in nationally recognized data sources to make visible how gaps in education and workforce infrastructure can produce compounding, system-wide consequences over time.

The purpose of these examples is to illuminate structural dynamics within nursing workforce development, rather than to predict individual student outcomes or generate causal estimates.

## EXAMPLE: BIOLOGY TEACHER IMPACT CALCULATION
### Assumptions and Sources

### 1. Average Annual Student Exposure: 30 students (conservative)

**Source:** National Center for Education Statistics. (2021). *Average class size in public K–12 schools, by school level, class type, and state: 2020–21.*

While average class size at a single point in time is lower (approximately 15–18 students per class at the secondary level), high school science teachers typically instruct multiple sections per year. This assumption reflects **conservative annual student exposure**, rather than per-section enrollment, and is used solely for illustrative purposes.

### 2. Teacher Tenure: 5 years

**Source:** Carver-Thomas, D., & Darling-Hammond, L. (2017). *Teacher turnover: Why it matters and what we can do about it.*

National data indicate median teacher tenure of approximately 5–7 years. A five-year assumption reflects a conservative estimate.

### 3. Students with Health Career Interest: ~12% (conservative)

**Sources (composite estimate):** National Student Clearinghouse Research Center. (2023). *Current term enrollment estimates.*

National Center for Education Statistics. (2022). *Fast facts: Degrees conferred by field of study.*

Across postsecondary systems, health-related fields account for approximately 6–7% of completed degrees, with higher proportions observed in current enrollment and declared majors. A 12%

assumption reflects a conservative estimate of student interest across secondary and postsecondary pathways.

### 4. Health-Interested Students Entering Nursing: ~30% (conservative)

**Sources:** U.S. Bureau of Labor Statistics. (2024a). *Registered nurses.* U.S. Bureau of Labor Statistics. (2024b). *Healthcare occupations.*

Registered nurses represent the **largest single occupation within the U.S. healthcare workforce**, and nursing consistently functions as one of the most common and accessible entry pathways into health careers. This assumption reflects nursing's relative prominence within healthcare occupations rather than a fixed proportion of total health professions enrollment.

## ILLUSTRATIVE CALCULATION

- 30 students/year × 5 years = 150 students total

- 150 students × 12% health career interest = 18 health-interested students

- 18 students × 30% nursing pathway selection = ~5–6 potential nurses

## INTERPRETIVE NOTE

These calculations intentionally rely on conservative assumptions. Actual workforce impacts may be higher in districts with robust health science pathways, strong postsecondary partnerships, or elevated local nursing workforce demand. The purpose of this illustration is to demonstrate how single points of failure in education infrastructure—such as the loss of a qualified science teacher—can generate multiplicative downstream effects, rather than simple one-to-one workforce losses.

These illustrative calculations are designed to clarify structural relationships within nursing workforce development and should not be interpreted as precise predictive models or causal estimates.

# References & Resources

## HOW TO USE THIS GUIDE

**For researchers:** Part 1 (Complete Bibliography) provides full APA citations for all sources referenced in this book.

**For practitioners:** Part 2 (Quick-Reference Guide) offers organizational context and entry points to workforce data, tools, and policy resources.

**For policymakers:** Together, these sections connect U.S. nursing workforce challenges to international best practices and federal policy levers.

## PART 1: COMPLETE BIBLIOGRAPHY

*All sources cited throughout The NEXUS
Nursing Framework™, arranged alphabetically.*

Carver-Thomas, D., & Darling-Hammond, L. (2017). *Teacher turnover: Why it matters and what we can do about it.* Learning Policy Institute. https://learningpolicyinstitute.org/product/teacher-turnover-report

Health Resources and Services Administration. (2021). *Health workforce projections*. U.S. Department of Health and Human Services. https://bhw.hrsa.gov/data-research/projecting-health-workforce-supply-demand

Health Workforce Australia. (2014). *Australia's future health workforce: Nurses detailed report*. Australian Government. https://www.health.gov.au/sites/default/files/documents/2021/03/nurses-australia-s-future-health-workforce-reports-detailed-report.pdf

International Council of Nurses. (2021). *Nursing leadership*. https://www.icn.ch/nursing-policy/nursing-leadership

International Council of Nurses. (2022). *Sustain and retain in 2022 and beyond: The global nursing workforce and the COVID-19 pandemic*. https://www.icn.ch/resources/publications-and-reports/sustain-and-retain-2022-and-beyond

International Labour Organization. (2020). *Care economy policy brief series*. https://www.ilo.org/global/topics/care-economy/lang--en/index.htm

International Labour Organization. (2022). *Care at work: Investing in care leave and services for a more gender-equal world of work*. https://www.ilo.org/publications/major-publications/care-work-investing-care-leave-and-services-more-gender-equal-world-work

National Academy of Medicine. (2021). *The future of nursing 2020–2030: Charting a path to achieve health equity*. The National Academies Press. https://doi.org/10.17226/25982

National Center for Education Statistics. (2021). *Average class size in public K–12 schools, by school level, class type, and state: 2020–21*. U.S. Department of Education. https://nces.ed.gov/surveys/ntps/

National Center for Education Statistics. (2022). *Fast facts: Degrees conferred by field of study*. U.S. Department of Education. https://nces.ed.gov/fastfacts/

National Student Clearinghouse Research Center. (2023). *Current term enrollment estimates*. https://nscresearchcenter.org/current-term-enrollment-estimates/

NHS England. (2023). *NHS long-term workforce plan.* https://www.england.nhs.uk/publication/nhs-long-term-workforce-plan/

Organisation for Economic Co-operation and Development. (2016). *Health workforce policies in OECD countries: Right jobs, right skills, right places.* OECD Health Policy Studies. OECD Publishing. https://doi.org/10.1787/9789264239517-en

Organisation for Economic Co-operation and Development. (2020). *Who cares? Attracting and retaining care workers for the elderly.* OECD Publishing. https://doi.org/10.1787/92c0ef68-en

Organisation for Economic Co-operation and Development. (2021). *Strengthening the frontline: How primary health care helps health systems adapt during the COVID-19 pandemic.* OECD Publishing. https://doi.org/10.1787/9a5ae6da-en

Strengthening Career and Technical Education for the 21st Century Act, Pub. L. No. 115–224, 132 Stat. 1563 (2018). https://www.congress.gov/bill/115th-congress/house-bill/2353

World Bank. (2018). *The human capital project.* World Bank Group. https://www.worldbank.org/en/publication/human-capital

World Bank. (2023). *Human capital index 2023 update.* World Bank Group. https://www.worldbank.org/en/publication/human-capital

World Economic Forum. (2020). *The future of jobs report 2020.* https://www.weforum.org/reports/the-future-of-jobs-report-2020

World Health Organization. (2020). *State of the world's nursing 2020: Investing in education, jobs and leadership.* https://www.who.int/publications/i/item/9789240003279

World Health Organization. (2021). *Global strategy on human resources for health: Workforce 2030.* https://www.who.int/publications/i/item/9789241511131

Wyoming Workforce Development Council. (n.d.). *About the Wyoming workforce system.* https://dws.wyo.gov/dws-division/councils-and-commissions/wwdc/

## PART 2: QUICK-REFERENCE
## GUIDE TO KEY ORGANIZATIONS

Specific reports and documents cited in this book are listed in Part 1. Organizational websites are provided here as entry points for additional tools, data, and policy resources.

This section offers organizational context and curated access points for practitioners, policymakers, educators, and researchers engaged in nursing workforce development. The organizations listed below are referenced throughout *The NEXUS Nursing Framework*™ and represent leading sources of global, national, and comparative workforce data and policy guidance.

### *Global Health Workforce Organizations*

**World Health Organization (WHO)** The World Health Organization leads global health workforce strategy and establishes international standards for nursing education, practice, and leadership. Its flagship nursing reports provide the most comprehensive global data on nursing supply, distribution, and policy trends.

### Key Resources

- *State of the World's Nursing 2020: Investing in Education, Jobs and Leadership*

- *Global Strategy on Human Resources for Health: Workforce 2030*

**Website:** https://www.who.int

**Focus Areas:** Global nursing workforce data, international standards, workforce planning frameworks

### International Council of Nurses (ICN)

The International Council of Nurses is the global voice of nursing, representing more than 27 million nurses worldwide through its network of national nursing associations. ICN advances nursing through advocacy, leadership development, and global workforce policy engagement.

**Key Resources**

- *Nursing Leadership* (policy and leadership frameworks)
- *Sustain and Retain in 2022 and Beyond*
- *ICN Workforce Forum reports and global position statements*

**Website:** https://www.icn.ch

**Focus Areas:** Nursing advocacy, professional standards, leadership development, workforce policy

### International Labour Organization (ILO)

The International Labour Organization examines care work as a cornerstone of economic development and gender equity. Its research focuses on labor conditions, workforce protections, and investment strategies for health and care workers globally.

**Key Resources**

- *Care Economy Policy Brief Series*
- *Care at Work: Investing in Care Leave and Services for a More Gender-Equal World of Work*

**Website:** https://www.ilo.org

**Focus Areas:** Care economy, labor rights, employment policy, gender equity in the health workforce

## ECONOMIC AND DEVELOPMENT ORGANIZATIONS

### *Organisation for Economic Co-operation and Development (OECD)*

The OECD conducts comparative analyses of health workforce policies across member countries, producing evidence-based guidance on workforce planning, education capacity, retention, and health system performance.

### Key Resources

- *Health Workforce Policies in OECD Countries: Right Jobs, Right Skills, Right Places*

- *Who Cares? Attracting and Retaining Care Workers for the Elderly*

- *Strengthening the Frontline: How Primary Health Care Helps Health Systems Adapt*

**Website:** https://www.oecd.org

**Focus Areas:** Comparative health workforce policy, retention strategies, health systems performance

### *World Bank*

The World Bank's Human Capital Project examines how investments in health and education drive long-term economic development. Its workforce research links nursing education infrastructure to broader development outcomes.

### Key Resources
- *The Human Capital Project*

- *Human Capital Index 2023 Update*

**Website:** https://www.worldbank.org
**Focus Areas:** Human capital development, health systems financing, workforce capacity building

### World Economic Forum (WEF)

The World Economic Forum analyzes global labor market trends and the future of work, including the transformation of healthcare roles. Its research situates nursing workforce development within broader economic, technological, and skills-based shifts.

**Key Resources**

- *The Future of Jobs Report 2020*

**Website:** https://www.weforum.org
**Focus Areas:** Future of work, digital transformation, workforce skills development

# U.S. FEDERAL AGENCIES AND POLICY ORGANIZATIONS

### Health Resources and Services Administration (HRSA)

HRSA, within the U.S. Department of Health and Human Services, administers federal nursing workforce investments and produces national workforce projections. HRSA plays a central role in funding nursing education, faculty development, and workforce distribution initiatives.

**Key Programs**

- Title VIII Nursing Workforce Development Programs

- Nurse Corps Loan Repayment Program
- Advanced Nursing Education Workforce Grants
- National Health Service Corps (NHSC)

## Key Resources
- *National health workforce projections*
- *Nursing workforce data and reports*

**Website:** https://www.hrsa.gov
**Focus Areas:** Nursing education funding, faculty development, workforce distribution, loan repayment

### National Academy of Medicine (NAM)

The National Academy of Medicine produces landmark consensus reports that shape U.S. nursing education, workforce policy, and scope-of-practice discussions. Its *Future of Nursing* series has guided national reform efforts for more than a decade.

## Key Resources
- *The Future of Nursing 2020–2030: Charting a Path to Achieve Health Equity*
- *The Future of Nursing: Leading Change, Advancing Health*

**Website:** https://nam.edu
**Focus Areas:** Nursing education transformation, health equity, leadership development, policy guidance

## ADDITIONAL FEDERAL RESOURCES
## REFERENCED THROUGHOUT THIS BOOK

**U.S. Department of Labor (DOL):** Workforce Innovation and Opportunity Act (WIOA), apprenticeships, O*NET occupational data

**U.S. Department of Education:** Perkins V Career and Technical Education Act, Pell Grants, and federal student aid programs

**Centers for Medicare & Medicaid Services (CMS):** Graduate Medical Education (GME) and reimbursement policies influencing clinical training capacity

**Bureau of Labor Statistics (BLS):** Nursing employment statistics and occupational projections

# INDEX

## A

Adult learners
  barriers and challenges, 76–81
  policy recommendations, 82–83
Accreditation requirements, 64,
  68, 69, 71, 105, 114, 115, 137
Apprenticeships, 31, 80, 84, 93, 94,
  115, 116, 125, 128, 129, 139, 144
Artificial intelligence (AI), 154,
  177, 184, 189, 194, 196

## B

Broadband access, 8, 18, 31,
  39, 67, 128, 192
Burnout, 7, 53, 106, 148, 149

## C

Clinical capacity
  educational challenges, 62–67, 70
  policy recommendations, 70
Community partnerships, 37, 189
Cross-sector collaboration
  framework overview, 135,
    140, 146, 147
  policy implications, 182, 189, 193

## D

Digital access, 9, 31, 39, 70, 80,
  128, 146, 156, 157, 167

## E

Educational capacity, 31, 39, 62, 79,
  104, 114, 128, 146, 155, 157

## F

Faculty shortages
  higher education challenges,
    62, 63, 70
  HRSA programs, 114
  policy recommendations, 70, 115
Faith-based organizations, 49,
    163, 179, 188, 197

## G

Global context, 2, 17, 18, 30, 36, 43,
    51, 62, 76, 86, 99, 108, 120, 134,
    135, 150, 160, 172, 181, 192

## H

Health Resources and Services
  Administration (HRSA)
  programs and funding, 107–117
  policy recommendations, 115

## I

Infrastructure, nursing workforce
  crisis overview, 17–20, 22, 23
  systemic solutions, 192, 193, 195, 201

## K

K–12 pathways
  framework overview, 35–41
  cross-sector integration, 133, 135–141

## N

National Academy of Medicine, 103
NEXUS Nursing Framework™
  conceptual overview, 29–34
  visual model, 33

## P

Perkins V
  overview and gaps, 75, 137, 141
  overview, 203

## S

Simulation and informatics, 25, 27,
    31, 39, 62, 64-67, 70
State innovation
  framework examples, 123
  policy recommendations, 129
Structural equity
  framework element, 48
  state applications, 128

## T

Title VIII (Nurse Education Act)
  overview and gaps, 97, 99–106
  HRSA administration, 108, 112, 116
  policy recommendations, 105–106
Transition to practice

## W

Workforce Innovation and
   Opportunity Act (WIOA)
   overview and gaps, 85–94
   cross-sector braiding, 136,
      137, 141, 145
   policy recommendations, 94

## Z

Zip code–based disparities, 196

# ABOUT THE AUTHOR

**Dr. Sherri Johnson** is a nationally recognized nurse leader, workforce development strategist, and health equity advocate with more than 25 years of experience across clinical practice, policy, and education. Her work focuses on building sustainable, student-centered pathways into nursing and healthcare careers, with a focus on expanding access and opportunity.

She has held senior leadership roles across multiple sectors and is the Founder of The Institute for Health and Social Equity, where she leads policy-informed initiatives advancing equitable workforce access across healthcare and STEM fields. Her work integrates research, community partnership, and policy levers to address persistent workforce gaps.

Dr. Johnson is a Fellow of the American Academy of Nursing and a frequent speaker and author on nursing leadership, workforce innovation, and equity. She is guided by the belief that zip code should never determine access—or opportunity.

www.ingramcontent.com/pod-product-compliance
Lightning Source LLC
Chambersburg PA
CBHW051613120626
46551CB00014B/1781